It's <u>Not</u> Your Fault You're FAT!

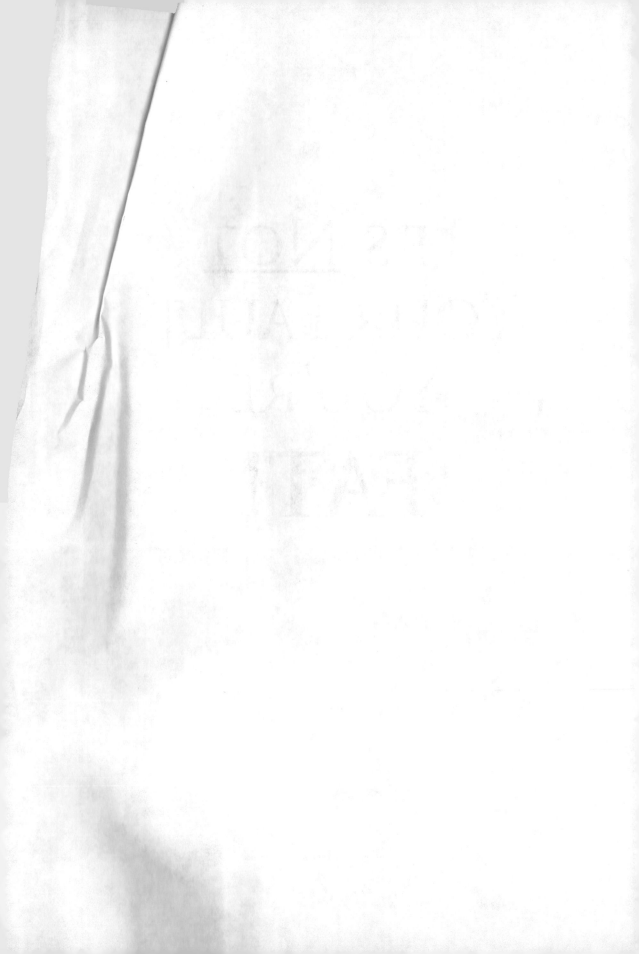

IT'S <u>NOT</u> YOUR FAULT YOU'RE FAT!

THE TOP 10 THINGS YOU <u>ABSOLUTELY</u> MUST KNOW TO LOSE WEIGHT FOR GOOD!

Dr. Sonia Kwapisinski, D. C.

with Dr. Edward Granat D.C.

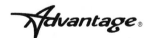

Published by Advantage, Charleston, South Carolina.
Member of Advantage Media Group.

ADVANTAGE is a registered trademark and the Advantage colophon is a trademark of Advantage Media Group, Inc.

Printed in the United States of America.

ISBN: 978-1-59932-194-3
LCCN: 2010904976

This publication is designed to provide accurate and authoritative information in regard to the subject matter covered. It is sold with the understanding that the publisher is not engaged in rendering legal, accounting, or other professional services. If legal advice or other expert assistance is required, the services of a competent professional person should be sought.

Most Advantage Media Group titles are available at special quantity discounts for bulk purchases for sales promotions, premiums, fundraising, and educational use. Special versions or book excerpts can also be created to fit specific needs.

For more information, please write: Special Markets, Advantage Media Group, P.O. Box 272, Charleston, SC 29402 or call 1.866.775.1696.

Visit us online at **advantagefamily**.com

INTRODUCTION

Let me begin by assuring you that this isn't one of those weight-loss books written by a stick-thin woman who has never struggled with her weight or with the ups and downs of dieting. I have been there myself and tried everything from the Atkins diet to the South Beach (which had pretty much nothing to do with a beach) to radioactive-green diet gum to eating only potatoes, and none of them worked. You name it, I've tried it, and with as little success as you have probably had.

I have helped my patients lose weight and realized that time and again, I was giving the same advice about their health and wellness. As a chiropractor and acupuncturist practicing holistic medicine for 10 years, I have helped many realize their true health potential. I decided to take it to heart for myself and share it with you. That's why I've decided to compile the <u>10 MUST-HAVE SECRETS</u> regarding weight loss for you. After all, isn't it about time you learned the truth about weight loss and your body?

In the following pages, I'm going to explain how your body really works and why that may be interfering with your weight-loss goals. Don't worry, I promise I won't boss you around or make you feel bad about your weight. I understand where you are coming from because I have been there myself and I've implemented the ideas and habits I am going to share with you. I have finally gotten to the bottom of my weight problems and made a change for the better (and healthier), and you can, too.

I managed to shed 32 pounds and kept them off for 15 years. It took me years, though, to learn what I am sharing with you. My weight came off in stages, but I will tell you ways to lose the weight fairly quickly and save you a lot of time and frustration.

For me, it was eating what was there. I had no instructions or directions when it came to food. So, in my mind, how could I possibly make the right choices?

BEFORE WE BEGIN

If you are a mother, you may cringe at how many adults' problems are blamed on their mothers. But, truly, the way we learn to eat as children does determine what kind of lifestyle we are going to have and whether or not we will be overweight. Our early childhood experiences will have determined much of our food habits, for good or bad. We are all 25 pounds heavier than we were 25 years ago! We can change that now!

You may already be fretting about your kids' bodies, especially if you are the mother of girls. Many of my patients first seek weight-loss advice when they start to see their daughters developing the same body type that they had when they were younger. These women remember the pain they felt as children and even more as adolescents who struggled to fit in despite being overweight. More than anything, they don't want their daughters to have to fight the same battles they have been fighting for so long. These women understand that if they can get their own health and weight under control, they will be able to help their daughters. It's like that old adage about putting your oxygen mask on before putting someone else's on for them: If you run out of air, you won't be any use to anyone else. In this case, until you have solved your own weight issues, you won't be able to help your daughter avoid having them for herself.

The good news about this for mothers is that you have the ability to have a positive effect on your daughters' lives with regards to weight! The relationship you have with food and are modeling for her will carry into her adulthood. If your preschool-age daughter catches you with your secret stash of Hershey's Kisses and you shoo her away, she won't really understand why, but she will know that you were eating and she got into trouble. She will also understand that food has power and can be used for more than satisfying hunger.

Because, as a mother, you are probably doing the bulk of the shopping, cooking and preparing of food, you can make a positive or negative impact on your children at each meal. Once you have worked through and implemented the ideas in this book, you will be able to bring them to your family and know that you are breaking the cycle of obesity that is gripping our whole society. You will be giving your children a gift of immeasurable value: a healthy start on life and, possibly more important, a healthy lifestyle that they can follow for good.

BACK TO MOM

It's always the mother's fault, isn't it? It may come as a relief to you that a good portion of your problem with weight can be linked back to your own mother. If you are like me, and most overweight people, you have internalized your feelings about your weight so that your identity is wrapped up in your weight. Whatever you are doing, whatever you accomplish, your thoughts will always go back to your size or how fat you feel in your outfit or what horrible mistake you made on your diet that day. We like to compare ourselves to the lowest weight we have ever been, which may not be the ideal weight for us right now.

Imagine if you could, just for a minute, that it's not your fault. Can you allow yourself to believe that? It's hard, I know. Most people who don't struggle with weight want to place all the blame on the fat people. They think that all fat people just sit around all day and eat junk food and don't care how they look. The truth is that most overweight people worry and think about food and weight nearly constantly. When I use the term "fat", please know I mean it in the nicest way. This is just the way I referred to myself for many years.

In the following chapters, let's take a look together at the 10 most important keys to weight loss so that you can change your health and your life for the better, and if you are a mom, or will be someday, you can make a positive impact on your children's lives.

We will discover:

• The role our genes play in our weight

• Our food history and its impact on our lifestyle

• The way we shop for food

• The way we think about food

• The way we choose our food

I am going to share with you what I have learned through a lifetime struggle with my own weight and through helping my patients get their lives and their weight under control. Some of the things I am going to tell you, you may already know – but maybe you haven't considered them in relation to weight loss. Others will be new information that I hope will put you on the road to weight-loss success!

TABLE OF CONTENTS

In this chapter, I will share the role our genes play in losing weight; how our eating history and habits affect our weight; as well as provide a rundown on how we digest food (enzymes, metabolism, digestion) and probiotics use.

In this chapter, we will discuss the importance of cleansing the body of internal toxins and outline the detox procedure, including its benefits and side effects.

It's impossible to lose weight (or keep it off) without learning what you should and shouldn't eat. In this chapter we'll discuss the importance of staying away from white flour, sugar, processed foods, hydrogenated oils, dairy, margarine, and even so-called diet foods.

There's no need to starve your body of the foods it wants (and craves). In this chapter, we will discuss what makes us crave certain foods and how to best handle those cravings. Plus, you will learn how to read your body's signals in order to get enough of the vitamins and minerals that are needed for optimum health and weight control.

Learning the right ways to buy food can make a big impact on your overall weight loss. This chapter will give the reader practical tips on shopping.

1

◇◇◇◇◇◇◇◇◇◇◇◇◇◇◇

THOU SHALT UNDERSTAND HOW THY BODY WORKS

We take our bodies for granted, even for all the worrying, fussing and primping we do on a daily basis. Most of us are far more concerned with our appearance than our health, and unless something is going wrong, we seem to give little thought to all the countless processes our cells are completing every day. We think about our digestion, maybe when our stomachs rumble either with hunger or with gas from overindulging on that all-you-can-eat lunch special, but do we really understand what is going on inside us and how our genetic makeup determines how our bodies will act and look? The answer is generally no, but we should!

IT'S ALL IN THE GENES
(YOUR MOTHER'S, THAT IS)

That's probably nicer than saying it's your mother's fault, but some of your weight problem may be partially as a result of your genes. We will discuss a bit later the other way our mothers made us fat (often by spoiling us with food!), but for now, let's take a look at the science behind weight and why some people just have an easier time maintaining a healthy weight while others struggle and fail.

If you were to look at a family portrait, what would you see? Would you see tall, slender people with thin wrists? If so, you probably would not be reading this book. Most of us who have weight problems have a genetic predisposition to being overweight, and it can be as simple as looking at a photograph to see where we get it. The old saying "the apple doesn't fall far from the tree" can be very true when it comes to weight. Of course, having obesity or even a little "chunkiness" in your family doesn't mean you are forever doomed to being overweight, but it does mean you will have to be more aware and conscious of your choices to overcome your genetic predisposition to store fat.

We, as a nation, are facing a crisis of obesity. According to the Centers for Disease Control (CDC), more than 34% of adults in the United States can be considered obese. With more and more children leading sedentary lifestyles and eating highly processed foods, these numbers will only grow in the future. Of course, genes take generations to change and develop, so these spikes in obesity rates cannot be entirely blamed on genetics. We will talk more a bit later about the type of diets and lifestyles we develop and how they carry from our childhood into our adulthood and bring the added pounds with them.

According to the Center for Human Nutrition, 66% of adults are overweight or obese, 16% of children and adolescents are overweight, and 34% are at risk of being overweight. By 2015, 75% of adults will be overweight and 41% will be obese.

If you are like me, you have tried every diet in the book only to either stay at the same weight, or, worse, to end up heavier than when you started. When I tried the Atkins diet, which seemed like a great idea at the time, I found myself feeling dizzy and faint and could barely remember how to tie my shoes. I pressed on, skipping all types of lovely carbohydrates in favor of a plate full of meat and cheese. When I finally gave in and ate a piece of bread, I realized that my skinny friends were eating the whole hamburger, bun and all, and not gaining weight. Why not me? It was infuriating!

The difference, in part, was genetics. My genetic makeup was obviously different than theirs. Current research is pointing geneticists in the direction of a gene that was probably necessary at one point in our ancestry to help people survive during times of famine. If you are heavy, and have fought that battle all your life, you are probably battling against a genetic predisposition to hold onto fat stores so that you will be able to survive when times are tough. In our society today, where food is plentiful and even overly abundant, these genes work against us rather than for us and leave us chunkier year after year. Researchers are working to isolate the single genes that affect and cause obesity, but for now, they understand that there is indeed a genetic component to being overweight. (See, it's your mother's fault after all!) However, you don't necessarily have to follow the path of your genes.

What you must understand, and tell yourself, is that you are not your weight or your mother's or anyone else's in your family. Because you are reading this book, you are ready and willing to make the changes you need to lose weight and take charge of your health and appearance. So, for once, give yourself a break and try to think clearly. If your mother wears glasses and your father wears glasses and you need to wear them, too, would you be upset or mad at yourself for needing glasses? Of course not! You would naturally accept the fact that poor eyesight runs in your family and you would take the necessary steps to correct it – in this case just by wearing glasses.

Now, take the same approach to your weight. Both of your parents are overweight and you have become an overweight adult. Your genes may have helped put you in this position, and now it's up to you to make the choice about what to do. You can either continue on the way you have been – indulging in the wrong kinds of foods, skipping exercise in favor of watching TV or spending time on the Internet, and not paying attention to your health. Or, you can take to heart my advice (and remember I have been where you are now) and make a change for the better. Because you are working against your genes, you won't be able to eat ice cream and sweets like your skinny friend (not if you want to lose weight), but you can attain and, more important, maintain a healthy weight and a great physical appearance.

FOOD HISTORY

When you think back to your childhood, what kinds of images come to mind? Days spent outside playing with friends and siblings? Maybe family gatherings or picnics? Vacations, big events and more probably pop into your mind very easily. What if I asked you about your food memories? Perhaps you have never considered taking an inventory of your food history to help put you on the path to weight loss, but I am not only suggesting it, I am insisting you do it right now!

Try to answer these questions as honestly as you can:

- Did you eat too much as a child, or never enough?

- Did you eat alone?

- Did you ever feel embarrassed by how much you ate?

- Were you able to stop eating when you were full, or were you encouraged to clean your plate?

- How was food used in your home (reward, love)?

- Was food pushed on you? Did you always celebrate with food?

Because we are both reminiscing and trying to unravel our food histories, I will share a couple of my own thoughts on the topic. When I was growing up, my mom stayed home with us kids when we were young. She prepared meals and did some baking until she went back to work. Then we ate take-out very frequently. A product of our time, eating out or bringing home take-out have become almost staples for today's busy families.

When my mother would put a great homemade dinner on the table, especially her "shake and bake" drumsticks, I would just eat and eat – as if someone was going to steal it from me if I didn't finish it first! One night in particular, I must have eaten a dozen drumsticks before anyone else could even sit down at the table; I literally couldn't stop eating them, they were that good! My mother was so upset with me because I had ruined dinner, but I had no little voice telling me to stop. I only had the urge to keep eating the food she had made. I ate everything that was there in front of me. I cleaned my plate, and everyone else's too.

I can remember going to the Red Lobster and getting the 30-shrimp special! Thirty shrimp! But I had no problem putting them away, and neither did my sister. Not only that, but we ate those delicious biscuits beforehand and washed it all down with unlimited refills of pop. I was probably around 12 years old at the time. My brother could handle eating anything – something about a skinny teenage boy's metabolism must have been at work there. My sister and I, on the other hand, gained more and more weight. We were like little piglets all lined up at the trough and we didn't know when to stop! I hope you are nodding your head in agreement at this point; otherwise I have shared an embarrassing childhood moment for nothing. I think you are, or you wouldn't be reading this book. Believe me, you are not alone. Millions of adults learned their bad eating habits in childhood and haven't broken them yet ("yet" being the key word).

Many of my patients have expressed to me that they used food to help with emotions even at a young age. They learned as kids to turn to food to find comfort, and that, coupled with their genetic predisposition, led them to being overweight as an adult. Knowing your food history and how you have come to use food for more than just fuel for your body will help you immeasurably as you begin this journey, which is about much more than a number on the scale. You can't go forward if you don't know and understand where you have been, so it makes sense to take a hard look at your own food history to determine what you are dealing with.

People who are just "naturally thin" use food for energy. This type of person eats only when she is hungry. Sometimes, she feels like eating ice cream; most of the time, she eats healthy food in moderate portions. She doesn't open the fridge when she is bored, tired, sad, frustrated, angry or upset. We will discuss attitude later in this book, but visualize that image for a moment and we will come back to it later.

DIGESTION: WHAT YOU NEED TO KNOW

Now that we have talked about your genes and about your food history, and before we get into what you should be eating, let's talk about how your digestive system works. It may not be the most glamorous part of the body, but your digestive system is as essential to your health as your heart or lungs, and if it is not functioning properly, it can affect everything from your energy levels to your blood pressure. Most of us don't give much thought to what goes on after we eat, unless we are suffering from indigestion or constipation, but it's good to know how your body processes food so that you can make better food choices and start feeling healthier right away.

Digestion occurs when enzymes that are created in the pancreas and excreted in digestive fluid break down our food and retrieve nutrients from it. Foods also contain enzymes, but many of these are killed during cooking and many of the over-processed foods that are a staple of our diets are devoid of enzymes.

The three main enzymes are:

- Amylase: responsible for digesting carbohydrates

- Protease: responsible for digesting proteins

- Lipase: responsible for digesting fats

Because our diets are lacking enzymes and we are constantly overloading our bodies with unhealthy foods, our organs (especially the pancreas) may be under extreme stress. The good news is that supplemental enzymes can be taken to help ease the burden on our digestive systems and break down our food better. Once the food is broken down the way it should be, we can get all the available nutrients from it and start reaping the benefits of weight loss, increased energy and improved health. Also, if you have been a sugar junkie at any time of your life, your normal gut flora (bacteria) that help with digestion are out of balance. You also may have an overgrowth of yeast. Taking a probiotic (lactobacillus/acidophilus) will help re-establish your good intestinal flora and get your colon back into balance. Check out www.itsnotyourfaultyourefat.com for a list of enzymes and my favorite probiotic.

ACCORDING TO DRS. ELLEN CUTLER AND JEREMY KASLOW IN **MICRO MIRACLES: DISCOVERING THE HEALING POWER OF ENZYMES**, "ENZYME THERAPY HELPS TAKE OFF UNWANTED POUNDS BY CORRECTING THE UNDERLYING DEFICIENCIES AND IMBALANCES THAT PREVENT ADEQUATE DIGESTION OF FOODS. OUR BODIES ARE BETTER ABLE TO ABSORB AND UTILIZE NUTRIENTS, SO THEY NO LONGER PROMPT US TO OVEREAT TO COMPENSATE FOR NUTRITIONAL SHORTFALLS. THEY ALSO STATE THAT, "ELIMINATING GRAINS CAN PROMOTE RAPID AND SIGNIFICANT WEIGHT LOSS."

It's all a lot to think about and understand, but it's a good start on our way to a healthier life and a more balanced one, too. Every part of our body – the genetics, the emotions, eating history and our digestion – are essential elements in our weight-loss success. If we don't take the time to understand these factors and what they have contributed to our weight gain, we won't be able to make the necessary changes to achieve our weight loss goals. It's all about getting our bodies to function optimally and as efficiently as possible.

2

_{◇◇◇◇◇◇◇◇◇◇◇◇◇◇◇◇}

THOU SHALT RID THY BODY OF TOXINS

You may have heard of a body detox and wondered what it is and whether it can really help you lose weight. There are many detoxification products on the market, all promising quick weight loss, some even promising to remove gigantic pieces of sludge from your colon. Take my advice, do not Google images of detoxifying unless you have a very strong stomach. The truth about a detox is hidden somewhere in all the hype, and a good detox program can help you get started on your way to a healthier life and a lower weight.

WHY DETOX?

What goes in must come out, right? Well, a lot of the junk we regularly put into our bodies never makes its way out. Physical signs that you might be ready for a detox program are constipation, bloating, fatigue, skin problems and indigestion. Don't wait for symptoms to appear, however – you can get the benefits of a good detox program even if you aren't suffering with any of those symptoms.

Basically, all the available methods have the same goal – to remove the multitude of toxins we have put into our bodies every day for years upon years. If you consider the amount of preservatives and artificial ingredients you ingest in a typical week of unhealthy eating, it's staggering. Even a simple snack from the vending machine in your office building probably has about 25 ingredients, many of them additives that are engineered to keep the food fresh for *months!* Those same additives stay in your body and wreak havoc in your digestive system.

You may not consider things like caffeine and alcohol to be toxins, but these substances have either a stimulating or depressing effect on the body. They need to be eliminated when you are seeking to achieve permanent and healthy weight loss. It almost goes without saying that if you smoke, you should quit. The evidence is irrefutable: Smoking causes cancer, lung disease, and a myriad of other health issues. You cannot achieve a healthy lifestyle if you are smoking. If you need help to quit smoking, you can always seek it from your physician or health care provider. (Acupuncture works great, by the way.) On the up side, a cleanse, or detoxification, will actually help you to quit because it will help flush the nicotine out of your system more quickly.

A detox program will also target the chemicals, pollutants and pesticides we are exposed to every day. In the next chapter, where we begin to discuss what we should be eating, we will spend some time talking about organically grown and hormone- free foods. For now, suffice it to say that even though we have become accustomed to having a wide variety of foods available nearly year round, the price has been high. Our genetically modified, pesticide-sprayed food is putting a strain on our digestive systems and causing all kinds of illnesses. Even when we think we are eating a healthy meal of chicken breast and salad, we may be ingesting large amounts of hormones and pesticides. A detoxification program will help to eliminate these pollutants and get our bodies ready for a healthier lifestyle.

NEW REPORT SHOWS A LINK BETWEEN ILL HEALTH AND TOXINS FOUND IN FOOD

A REPORT RELEASED BY THE PESTICIDE ACTION NETWORK NORTH AMERICA AND COMMONWEALTH FINDS THAT AMERICANS CAN EXPERIENCE UP TO 70 DAILY EXPOSURES TO RESIDUES OF A CLASS OF TOXIC CHEMICALS KNOWN AS PERSISTENT ORGANIC POLLUTANTS – POPS – THROUGH THEIR DIETS ALONE.

THE REPORT, "NOWHERE TO HIDE: PERSISTENT TOXIC CHEMICALS IN THE U.S. FOOD SUPPLY," ANALYZES CHEMICAL RESIDUE DATA COLLECTED BY THE FOOD AND DRUG ADMINISTRATION (FDA) AND FINDS PERSISTENT CHEMICAL CONTAMINANTS IN ALL FOOD GROUPS – FROM BAKED GOODS AND MEATS TO FRESH FRUITS AND VEGETABLES.

EXPOSURE TO POPS HAS BEEN LINKED TO SERIOUS DISEASE AND DEVELOPMENTAL DISORDERS, INCLUDING BREAST AND OTHER TYPES OF CANCER, IMMUNE SYSTEM SUPPRESSION, NERVOUS SYSTEM DISORDERS, REPRODUCTIVE DAMAGE, AND DISRUPTION OF HORMONAL SYSTEMS.

After a detox program, most people report increased energy and a feeling of overall lightness that is a result of the dislodging of "gunk" from the colon. Your intestinal system is like the pipes in your home. Just as pipes get congested and move more slowly, so will your colon. Once the intestines are clogged, it is nearly impossible to absorb the nutrients in your food. It's time to clean out the debris that has built up over time. After a detox and then following a healthy diet, you can expect to have a bowel movement after every meal. Yes, every meal!

HOW DO I DETOXIFY?

You may be ready to get to work on detoxifying or you might be worried about what lies ahead for you. If you are truly ready to get a fresh start on a healthy lifestyle, detoxifying is for you. There are many ways to flush the toxins from your body, some extreme and some not worth your time. We will look at the major ones that are helpful and healthful:

- Herbal cleansing

- Juice fasting

- Raw foods/vegetarian

- Colonics and enemas (yes, really!)

- Supplements (such as natural fiber called psyllium, or apple pectin). A great product that's easy and gentle is called Experience, found on www.itsnotyourfaultyourefat.com.

HERBAL CLEANSING

If you walk into your neighborhood drugstore, surf the Internet, or watch TV for any amount of time, you will encounter an advertisement for herbal cleansing. Herbal detoxification seems to be the most popular diet aid these days, and although it is very popular right now, it has been around for a long time and can be very effective in ridding the body of toxins and getting a good start on your new healthy lifestyle.

These herbal cleansing formulas generally have a few characteristics in common: They are usually taken for weeks to months; they are made up of several supplements; and they use a laxative component and a replenishing component to get the job done. Herbal supplement cleansing formulas are usually taken in the morning and the evening and the two (or more) components work together to loosen the contents of the colon and move it along, while replacing any nutrients lost during the process. I have my favorite products listed on my Web site at www.itsnotyourfaultyourfat.com.

WHAT TO EXPECT WITH AN HERBAL CLEANSE

With a gentle herbal cleanse, such as my favorite, Experience, you can expect to have a major bowel movement in the morning. Some stronger cleanses can affect you throughout the day, so don't start one if you have to be on a train all day or be outside at your kid's soccer game with only a porta-potty nearby. You should be having frequent bowel movements and be feeling less bloated and full within the first few days.

It's also very important to stay hydrated while doing any type of cleanse. If your body is voiding more than usual, you are losing more fluids than usual and you need to replenish what is lost as well as keep yourself well-hydrated. You should also eat lightly and avoid heavy or processed foods while doing a cleanse so that your body isn't working against itself. Of course, in the next few chapters, we will be seriously changing your eating habits – before you know it you will be avoiding those sugary processed foods you think you can't live without!

JUICE FASTING

Fasting has long been a part of many cultures throughout the world. Many religions include fasting as part of their rituals, whether as simple as abstaining from food for a day or going without for up to a month. The basic idea of a fast is that by depriving the body of input for a day (or more), your internal systems will be forced to purge themselves of toxins. Juice fasts offer more nutrition than a strict fast and last from one to three days. Before embarking on a juice fast, it is important to consult with your doctor or health care provider if you suffer from diabetes or hypoglycemia, or if you regularly take prescription medication, as the drop in food, and, therefore, blood sugar could have an adverse effect.

About a week before a juice fast, you should start to wean yourself from caffeine and alcohol and limit sugar, wheat, dairy and animal protein. Adopting a healthy diet of organic vegetables and protein before beginning the fast will help you avoid such common and annoying side effects as headaches and fatigue.

You can't just share your kid's Juicy Juice or get a container of OJ to do a juice fast; you have to use freshly juiced fruits and vegetables. The do-it-yourself method provides the freshest ingredients and most nutrients, but if you don't have access to a juicer and have a health food store nearby, you could rely on it for a supply of fresh, organic juice for the fast. Plan to consume between 32 and 64 ounces of the juice throughout the day while on the fast, along with at least six glasses of water. Green vegetables may not sound like a good ingredient for juice, but the chlorophyll in dark-green, leafy veggies, plus their high vitamin and nutrient content, make them a great addition to a juice fast.

The basis for a juice fast is to give your digestive system both a rest and a boost. The rest comes from having only liquids go through the colon for a day or more, and the boost from the presence of super-healthy plant enzymes that help replenish the digestive enzymes we are all lacking these days. Once you have finished your fast, you should slowly return to a regular, healthy diet. Juice fasts increase energy and improve moods and can jump-start your new healthy lifestyle. Juices can include vegetables such as carrots; broccoli; spinach, kale and other dark-green leafy vegetables; celery; and dandelion. Fruits can include apples, oranges, grapefruit, and berries. No grapes! Juices should be 80% green, 20% remaining colors. Spinach and celery make a great base for the green. Carrots and apples are great for flavor. If you don't want to fast, just use the juice as part of your regular routine, preferably in the morning.

BENEFITS OF A DETOX DIET

ACCORDING TO THE NEW DETOX DIET, BY DR. ELSON HAAS, JUICE FASTING OR JUICING FOR THREE TO FOUR DAYS IS GENERALLY SAFE AND VERY VERSATILE WITH SEVERAL HEALTH BENEFITS. JUICING BREAKS DOWN CIRCULATING OR STORED CHEMICALS BY REDUCING CALORIC INTAKE TO THE POINT WHEREIN OUR ORGANS CAN SPEND MORE TIME DETOXIFYING OUR BODY (I.E. COLON, KIDNEYS, LIVER, LUNGS, SINUSES, AND SKIN), THUS ELIMINATING WASTE PRODUCTS, IMPROVING CELLULAR NUTRITION AND INCREASING OXYGENATION. THOSE IN POOR HEALTH SHOULD UNDERGO MEDICAL SUPERVISION WHILE FASTING.

RAW FOODS/VEGETARIAN DETOXIFICATION

Inherent in all the detoxification methods is the idea that we are all full of pollutants, whether from additives or from sugars, starches and fats. We have cultivated a taste (culturally and individually) for the unhealthy foods we are surrounded with. If we love french fries and soda, it is very hard to get used to eating leafy greens and fresh fruits even though we were designed to eat those very things.

When I was a kid, my mom would come home from grocery shopping with a case of pop and a box of Flakys. You may not remember them, but I loved them, all the sugar you could ever want in the form of a puff pastry filled with fake cream and red goop. I ate the entire box (six to be exact). My mother then wised up and started to buy two boxes a week. Now, was I naturally inclined to eat those foods? No, of course not! But I developed a taste for them (oh, did I) and I loved them and all kinds of unhealthy and sugary foods. I taught my taste buds to crave sweets.

A detox program can effectively break that addiction to sugar. After purging the body of harmful foods and pollutants, you will find that your cravings are nearly gone. Of course, you will still have to find ways to break the emotional habits that lead you to eat, but a good detox program can help break the physical dependence and preference for these horrible foods.

The raw foods or vegetarian detox is a great way to break the cycle of our modern eating habits. Simply eating raw or slightly cooked vegetables and fruits for every meal for up to a week can radically change your body and your digestive system for the better. The healthy plant enzymes, which are still alive and kicking in raw veggies, will replenish your digestive system. The infusion of fresh, healthy food will help to reorient your body and your taste buds away from the sweet and sugary or salty and fatty foods most of us have become accustomed to eating.

After a week on a vegetarian detox, it would be hard to even imagine consuming a fast-food meal!

COLONICS: NOT FOR THE FAINT OF HEART

You may have heard of celebrities getting "colonics." They are often in fashion with actresses and models, but they are an ancient way of cleaning out the body's plumbing, so to speak, and aren't a new fad by any means. Colonics are basically the introduction of water into the colon through the rectum. You cannot give yourself a colonic; you would see a specialist who would administer the process for you. An enema can be done at home and involves the same principle of adding water to the colon, but deals only with the lower portion of the colon, not the entire length.

Colonics are basically safe for most people and, although they sound pretty gross, are actually not that bad. A tube is inserted into the rectum and introduces water into the colon to encourage built-up fecal matter to evacuate. The waste is removed through the tube, so that there is no smell or interaction with the fecal matter. Once the procedure is over (about 45 minutes later) the person would sit on the toilet to allow any remaining fluid or waste to leave the body.

Proponents of colonics praise them for their ability to detoxify the body and help with digestive problems as well as abdominal pain, rashes and other illnesses.

We are all full of crap – literally! Detoxing is all about eliminating the junk we have absorbed and ingested, and that is so appealing to those of us who know that we haven't taken our health seriously!

Once you have cleaned it all out, you can start on the road to real health.

Easy: Herbal cleanse

Medium: Juice fast

Gutsy Yet Painless: Colonic

3

_{◇◇◇◇◇◇◇◇◇◇◇◇◇◇}

THOU SHALT LEARN WHAT TO EAT

Let's be honest, we all know what we shouldn't be eating, right? Well, sort of. We often mean well, but don't always realize the unhealthy choices we're making. When I used to run to the drive-through and pick up some fries and a greasy burger for lunch, I knew it wasn't healthy. Even as I worried and complained about the weight I was gaining and the clothes that didn't fit, I knew that the food I was eating wasn't good for me. In fact, if I hadn't changed my eating habits, I would not only be heavier today, I would be on the road to disease!

There was a time when I asked my mother to buy me Lean Cuisine frozen dinners, thinking they were healthy. She responded, "How many of those are you going to eat? Three?" Turns out frozen dinners aren't good for you, after all. Sticking to fresh foods is much better whenever possible.

We all carry our food histories with us from childhood into adulthood, but at this point we need to pass on the pasta and start eating healthy food that will fuel our bodies and nourish us. I think back to grade school, when I used to go skiing with a friend. Now, she was a champion skier and I could barely stay up on my skis, but I loved our weekly trips because we always went to Kentucky Fried Chicken before heading up to the mountain. That was seriously my favorite part! I even loved the bright green, mayo-laden coleslaw that was the "vegetable" for my meal. After about one or two runs down the hill, we would go into the chalet for more fries!

When I was a kid, it was my parents' responsibility to make sure I understood what kinds of food were healthy and which weren't. They also should have taught me (and yours should probably have taught you) that food is simply fuel for our bodies, not an answer to problems or emotional issues. Up until this point, we have talked about the things we really can't control: our genes, our eating history and our basic biology. But now you really can take charge and get a fresh start when it comes to your weight and your health. It's time to put away those habits we've had since we were kids and work with our genes – it's time to learn to eat.

THE LOWDOWN ON OUR FOOD SUPPLY

Before we start talking about making changes in our eating habits, let's talk a bit about the food that is available on store shelves. You may think that going all-fresh is best – and it may be. The problem is that even fresh fruits and vegetables may not be as good for you today as they once were.

In our attempt to make everything bigger and better (including our food), our society has managed to ruin some good – no, I mean great – things. The first thing we've done is ruin the soil in which our crops are grown.

Good soil is the basis for a healthy life. Unless the soil in which we grow our food is made up of 45% minerals, it cannot grow the vitamin/mineral-rich foods we need. According to researcher Dr. William Albrecht of the University of Missouri, "mineral-deficient soil is one of the original sources of disease in the world today." He concludes that until we can replenish our soil, the human race will continue to battle a myriad of ongoing health concerns.

All you have to do is compare today's fresh fruits and vegetables with those from 20, 30 or 40 years ago. Who hasn't noticed the deterioration of taste and quality through the years? If you haven't noticed a difference, you definitely need to read further. Remember those juicy red apples you picked from your grandparents' backyard apple tree when you were a kid? The odds are that you haven't found an apple tasting that good in years. How about those red ripe tomatoes your mother grew in her garden? Found anything even close to those in recent years? The odds are you're shaking your head right now, saying, "Yeah, why doesn't food taste as good these days?" The answer is: the soil it's grown in.

As farmers added more and more pesticides to their crops to keep them free of bugs and other natural damage, the soil they used became more and more depleted of its natural minerals.

In order for farmers to grow more resistant plants, the crops we glean our food from today are nothing more than bioengineered plants that contain less than half of the nutrients the same fruit or vegetable did when we were children.

WHY TRACE MINERALS ARE IMPORTANT

Poor soil content is responsible for a lack of much-needed trace minerals in the foods we eat today. The human body requires a certain amount of selenium, boron, chromium and more to work properly. Derived from plants (which absorb them from the soil), these trace minerals aren't as abundant in the plants and animals we eat as they once were, and this is causing some serious health problems like:

- A deficiency in Vitamin B12 – without enough cobalt available in our food, your body cannot make B12 in the right amounts.

- Tachycardia – potassium, an important trace mineral, helps keep the heart pumping regularly and without it, this important muscle can't beat at the proper intervals.

- An inability to detoxify the blood – trace minerals such as zinc, selenium, sulfur and iron all help the liver to flush out toxins from the body. Without the proper amounts of each of these important minerals, the liver can become sluggish, becoming unable to repair damaged tissues.

- An inability to fight infections – the most important ingredient in a plant is its enzymes, which require a variety of trace minerals in order to thrive. Without the right amount (and kinds of) enzymes in the plants we eat, our immune systems are unable to fight infection.

Our body needs all of the 90-plus known trace elements in order to thrive. Missing just a few can cause irreparable harm to each and every organ that keeps us alive and well.

The only real solution to this problem is to buy organic produce. While they may not look as pretty and perfect as their bioengineered counterparts, organic fruits and veggies contain the right amount of vitamins, minerals and nutrients necessary to keep our bodies running smoothly so that we can finally lose the weight we need to.

THE CHEMICALIZATION OF OUR FOOD SUPPLY

The deterioration of our food supply, and the subsequent obesity crisis it has caused, doesn't stop with our nutrient-poor soil. Not only have we over-treated the earth, but also we've over-chemicalized our foods – all in the quest of making them last longer and look better. All it's really done is make us sicker – and fatter!

According to the National Cancer Institute in the SEER Cancer Statistics Review, cancer has increased since 1975. Why? Because 50 years ago, people ate fresh, whole foods (including butter); processed foods weren't available. No chemicals, no pesticides, no preservatives, no jumbo size.

Today, however, our diet is rich in bleached, refined, preserved, pasteurized, sterilized, hydrogenated, artificially colored, salted, sugared and enriched foods, filled with hundreds of artificial ingredients and chemicals designed to make them taste better, look better and last longer on the shelf! Plus, despite spending billions of dollars every year on diet and exercise aids, Americans grow bigger and bigger with each passing year. See a coincidence between the chemicalization of our food and our expanding waistlines, buttocks and thighs? I do!

Now, if you think I'm trying to get out of taking responsibility for my weight problems, I'll admit it – I am! But the truth is that while we each do have some responsibility to bear for our weight, it isn't solely a problem about proportion sizes or an inability to say no. My weight and your weight also have a lot to do with the foods available for us to eat!

THE GOOD, THE BAD AND THE UGLY

When it comes to dieting, we have tried it all, haven't we? I know I tried every crazy diet that was in fashion until I realized that none of those fads would really get to the heart of the problem and help me lose weight.

I tried Weight Watchers and only lasted a day – one day! I couldn't believe I had to stand up in a room full of people and get weighed in like a cow! I sucked it up, got weighed and headed home ready to implement the plan. After only the first day, I was finished with weighing and measuring everything, and I was starving! Plus, my brother and sister were having a field day with the harassing comments about my "diet"! That was enough for me; I sneaked down to the kitchen and ate my way through a pound of thinly sliced salami. At one point I even stuck my finger down my throat to make myself throw up, but it didn't work. Lucky for me. (I don't recommend it.)

I knew, basically, what not to eat, but what should I eat? I mean, breaking your mental and physical addiction to sugary and fatty foods can be like quitting smoking or getting sober. A drug addict can stop taking drugs; a smoker can just eliminate cigarettes. A person has to eat – there is no choice but to learn how to eat if you want to be healthy and lose weight. You can't eliminate your eating habit; you must change it drastically.

You can eat healthy and delicious foods and lose weight – really! The key is to understand what foods are really good for you, and you may be surprised to find out that diet foods are not! Many so-called diet or low-fat foods are full of artificial ingredients, empty calories or sodium that are added to replace the taste of the fat or flavorings that have been taken out. Honestly, a salad dressing should have a little oil in it, right? Well, oil is fat and as we will see there are good fats and bad fats, but if you take out all the fat, what will replace it? Usually sugar. The same with cookies; if they are low-fat, something needs to take the place of the fat that should be in a baked good, and if you are getting those goodies off the grocery shelves, watch out! Hydrogenated oils and preservatives are the enemy of our intestinal systems. Diet foods also leave us wanting more, so often we consume more of these low-fat impersonators because we think it can't hurt to have two more cookies if they are low-fat, right? Well, it can!

Our bodies are not made to process the amount and variety of artificial food products we are ingesting. It really is no surprise that obesity levels are rising at such an alarming rate when a good portion of our collective diet is made up of processed foods. Many diets will ask you to eliminate fats, but a healthy fat like olive oil (extra virgin is best) can be easily digested and doesn't put the kind of stress on your body that the multitude of artificial and engineered products will. A pat of butter is healthier than the equivalent amount of margarine because it is made from natural ingredients (cream, salt) that your body knows how to digest. Margarine is full of hydrogenated oil, which clogs the pipes, starts to rot, and can give you colon cancer. As for diet sodas, they are the enemy! Seriously, avoid diet sodas like the plague; they are loaded with sodium, which can increase your blood pressure. And, they often just activate your taste buds with their sweetness, but since your body isn't getting any calories, it puts you on the prowl for more and more sweets! The chemicals and sweeteners that make them "diet" are neurotoxic. This means they are toxic to your nervous system (nerves and brain). They can impair your judgment as well as your digestion, make you depressed and hinder your immune system. I used to love Diet Coke when I was in college in my early 20s, but all it got me was a kidney stone at age 21! But, that's where I landed after making a meal out of Diet Coke and popcorn so many nights with my girlfriends. Funny how no one in the hospital ever said anything to me about diet. They just told me to lose weight. (Thanks a lot!)

Luckily, I've learned a lot since then about how to eat, what to eat and what to avoid completely. I have been able to lose the weight I have struggled with since childhood, not only by eliminating bad food, but also – and maybe more important – by introducing super-healthy foods into my diet.

THE BIG THREE

Lean, Organic Protein

The typical American's diet consists of way too many over-processed carbohydrates and only a small amount of the protein we need for good health. Protein is essential for building and maintaining muscle, and for the repair of tissues. Our bodies need protein for the health of our bones, cartilage, skin and blood, but we are unable to store protein in our bodies. All the protein we need must come from our diets.

Protein-only, or protein-heavy diets were all the rage just a decade ago – believe me, I remember. People were losing huge amounts of weight by eating fatty, greasy meats, cheeses and eggs – and nothing else. I will admit I bought into this craze, just as I have many others. After this fad went out of style, we sort of lost our interest in protein, but we should pay close attention to this important component to lose weight and maintain that loss.

Adults need 46 to 56 grams of dietary protein each day, as part of a healthy and well-rounded diet. Your protein intake should come from lean meats, poultry and especially fish, which is so healthy and chock-full of important omega-3 vitamins. Look for organic meats first, then natural, and wild fish because these won't have growth hormones or other additives that we don't need and shouldn't be ingesting.

Eggs can be an important part of protein intake when you are dieting. The humble egg has gotten a bad rap in the cholesterol department, but eggs are actually very healthy and a great source of protein. A large egg contains 213 milligrams of cholesterol, just 100 milligrams shy of the recommended dietary cholesterol for a day. But, as researchers are learning, the body might not directly absorb cholesterol found in eggs, and the nutrition benefits far outweigh the cholesterol. Eggs are a great source of protein, Vitamins A, B-6, B-12 and folic acid, which are all good for your heart. Again, when buying eggs, try to buy locally or look for a good organic brand.

Organic Fresh Fruits and Vegetables

The cornerstone of a healthy diet must be fresh vegetables and a little fruit (those low on the glycemic index). Nutrient-rich, low in calories and flavorful, fresh produce will be your new friend, and once you have kicked your refined sugar habit you will find your taste buds in tune with nature's desserts. Buy fresh and organic whenever possible. Avoid canned vegetables, because they are heavily salted and much of their nutritional value is lost in canning. I would totally avoid canned fruits as they are often floating in sugar. Also, avoid eating anything from a can or plastic bottle as the added chemicals and hormones wreak havoc on your system.

Vegetables also provide dietary fiber, which regulates your digestive system and gives you energy. Veggies are filling and healthy, which will help you lose weight and increase your energy levels. You won't be running on a sugar high, only to crash when those simple carbohydrates poop out on you. Energy from the complex carbs in vegetables is with you for the long haul.

ORGANIC FRUITS AND VEGETABLES HAVE A HIGHER NUTRIENT CONTENT

ACCORDING TO A RECENT STUDY RELEASED BY RESEARCHERS AT THE UNIVERSITY OF CALIFORNIA, ORGANICALLY GROWN TOMATOES CONTAIN 79 TO 90 PERCENT MORE MICRONUTRIENTS THAN THEIR NONORGANIC COUNTERPARTS. THIS IS GOOD NEWS FOR THOSE TRYING TO MAINTAIN A HEALTHY DIET, EXCEPT FOR THE FACT THAT STATISTICS SHOW THAT TOMATOES ARE THE SECOND MOST-ALTERED CROP IN THE U.S. TO DATE

Healthy Fats

You might be thinking that the term "healthy fats" is an oxymoron, and you wouldn't be alone. A common thought among dieters is that we should eliminate all fats from our diets, but that isn't a truly healthy option. As we discussed earlier, many low-fat foods are actually chock-full of preservatives, artificial fillers and sugar that are trying desperately to take the place of the fat necessary for adding flavor to our food. But, as all of us tried to take the fat out of our foods, we seemed to be adding the fat to our waistlines. It's not just about the amount of fat you ingest; it's the type of fat, as well.

Healthy fats are the monounsaturated fats that supply our bodies with the essential fatty acids necessary for every system in our bodies, from our brains to our cardiovascular system to the surfactant in our lungs. We need fats, but we don't need hydrogenated oils, they just build up in our intestinal system and can cause cancer. Opt for extra-virgin olive oil or grape seed oil and you will be well on your way to weight loss and better health.

Another great reason to consume olive oil (extra-virgin is best):

ACCORDING TO THE AUGUST 12 ISSUE OF THE JOURNAL OF THE AMERICAN MEDICAL ASSOCIATION, FOLLOWING A MEDITERRANEAN DIET AND INCREASING LEVELS OF EXERCISE WERE ASSOCIATED WITH A LOWER RISK OF ALZHEIMER'S DISEASE. THIS DIET IS HIGH IN FRUITS, VEGETABLES, LEGUMES, FISH AND OLIVE OIL AS THE MAIN SOURCE OF MONOUNSATURATED FAT.

One way to keep healthy oils in your diet is to skip the premade salad dressings and opt for oil and vinegar or freshly squeezed lemon and lime that you put on yourself. The health and flavor benefits of simple olive oil and balsamic vinegar will far outweigh (no pun intended) the ease of using a prepared dressing. Another advantage to using oil and vinegar is that you won't be introducing sugars and extra carbs into your healthy salads.

A WORD ABOUT CARBOHYDRATES

White pasta, cookies, white rice and cake are all to be avoided. In fact, if you really want to lose weight, you should try to avoid any simple carbohydrates. White flour, white sugar and over-processed carbohydrates will foil your plans for losing weight time after time.

Sugary treats are also evil. I know, you're saying, "I can't stop!" You can! Once you give your body what it really needs, you won't crave the sweets anymore.

The big problems with not only sweets, but also bread, cereal, crackers, juices and pop, is that they usually contain fructose, a sugar. And all sugars are not made alike. Calories in do not equal calories out. That's why counting calories typically fails. Where the calories come from matters. Fructose gets stored as fat much more easily than glucose, for example. Fructose also depresses the hormone leptin, which tells you when you're full. If leptin stops working, you will continue to overeat, store fat and gain weight. Fructose is hidden in almost every processed food. This is the BIGGEST problem of them all. We are being tricked. You buy some whole-grain bread and you think you're doing the right thing? Read the label. The bread is very likely to contain fructose. You also need to be watchful of fruit, as it also contains fructose. Eat only 1 serving of fruit per day. Take a look at the chart extracted from Dr. Mercola's website to see how much fructose is in each fruit. Dr. Mercola recommends eating 15 g of fructose per day or less. Note: Do not eat any dried fruit. The sugars are highly concentrated so just avoid it all together.

FRUIT	SERVING SIZE	GRAMS OF FRUCTOSE
Limes	1 Medium	0
Lemons	1 medium	0.6
Cranberries	1 cup	0.7
Passion Fruit	1 medium	0.9
Prune	1 medium	1.2
Apricot	1 medium	1.3
Guava	2 medium	2.2
Date (Deglet Noor Style)	1 medium	2.6
Cantaloup	1/8 of med. melon	2.8

FRUIT	SERVING SIZE	GRAMS OF FRUCTOSE
Rasberries	1 cup	3.0
Clementine	1 medium	3.4
Kiwifruit	1 medium	3.4
Blackberries	1 cup	3.5
Star fruit	1 medium	3.6
Cherries, Sweet	10	3.8
Strawberries	1 cup	4.0
Cherries, sour	1 cup	4.0
Pineapple	1 slice (3.5" x .75")	4.0
Grapefruit, pink or red	1/2 medium	4.3
Boysenberries	1 cup	4.6
Tangerine/mandarin orange	1 medium	4.8
Nectarine	1 medium	5.4
Peach	1 medium	5.9
Orange (naval)	1 medium	6.1
Papaya	1/2 medium	6.3
Honeydew	1/8 of med. melon	6.7
Banana	1 medium	7.1
Blueberries	1 cup	7.4
Date (Medjool)	1 medium	7.7
Apple (composite)	1 medium	9.5
Persimmon	1 medium	10.6
Watermelon	1/16 med. melon	11.3
Pear	1 medium	11.8
Raisins	1/4 cup	12.3
Grapes, seedless (green or red)	1 cup	12.4
Mango	1/2 medium	16.2
Apricots, dried	1 cup	16.4
Figs, dried	1 cup	23.0

A diet high in sugar and grains will increase fat that gets stored in your body. This will increase leptin, and over time, if there is too much leptin, your body becomes de-sensitized to it and you become leptin-resistant, just like you can become insulin resistant, which we will discuss shortly. If you become leptin- resistant, your body does not know when to stop eating, therefore it remains hungry and stores more fat.

ACCORDING TO DR. DAVID LUDWIG, WHO TREATS CHILDHOOD OBESITY AT CHILDREN'S HOSPITAL BOSTON, SAYS ONE PROBLEM IS THAT HIGHLY PROCESSED CARBOHYDRATES AND REFINED SUGARS ARE CAUSING HORMONAL CHANGES THAT "DRIVE HUNGER, CAUSE OVEREATING, AND INCREASE THE RISK OF DIABETES AND HEART DISEASE."

According to the latest research out of Johns Hopkins University and research by Dr. Patrick Quillin, director of nutrition for Cancer Treatment Centers of America, sugar feeds cancer cells. We all have cancer cells in our bodies that are broken down by a healthy immune system. If you have any type of disease or health issue, <u>ELIMINATE ALL REFINED SUGARS!</u> Avoid white sugar and white flour. Also avoid milk. It produces mucus, which also feeds cancer cells, according to a March 2009 John Hopkins University newsletter.

When we eat simple carbs such as sugar and white flour, our bodies get an instantaneous burst of energy that may pick us up for a bit or lighten our mood or relax us – but the effects are short-lived and we are often back in the pantry looking for more sugar to keep us in that euphoric state just a little bit longer. Remember that potato-chip slogan, "You can never eat just one"? Well, there was some truth to that ad: most of us can't eat just one – one leads to another and another, and pretty soon we are sitting on the sofa covered in chip crumbs and filled with regret. Eliminating these foods from your diet can be tough at first – their hold on us can border on addictive – but once the cycle is broken and you are able to choose better snacks, you will be on your way to permanent weight loss. I suggest having some boiled eggs in the fridge, cut raw veggies, nuts/seeds and some avocado handy for when you come home starving. Eating a handful of nuts or an egg will prevent a serious binge in front of the fridge. I sometimes would eat a tablespoon of real peanut butter to curb my hunger. It worked like a charm.

The whiter the food, the worse it will be for your waist!

WHAT IS A SUGARHOLIC TO DO?
IF YOU NEED SOMETHING SWEET, USE THE FOLLOWING:
STEVIA
ORGANIC RAW HONEY

AVOID AT ALL COSTS:

FRUCTOSE
SUCROSE
SPORTS DRINKS/ ENERGY DRINKS
STORE-BOUGHT FRUIT JUICES
SODA POP
ARTIFICIAL SWEETENERS

THE FACTS ABOUT THE GLYCEMIC INDEX

All of this leaves us to discuss the glycemic index in order to get the right balance of foods and give your body a boost at losing weight.

Maybe you have been hearing a lot about this unique eating plan, but still don't quite understand how it works. Well, I'm going to tell you.

I have found this simple plan to be one of the best in the fight against growing wider instead of wiser as we age. And it's easy to incorporate into your eating plan. All it really entails is taking a good hard look at the ways in which the foods you eat may be affecting your blood glucose levels – and ultimately your weight.

Every time you eat high-glycemic foods such as breads, pastas and baked goods (all the tasty stuff), your blood sugar rises and falls quickly. That's why you feel full fast and hungry again even faster, and tend to snack between meals with – you guessed it – another high-glycemic food. This is a recipe for gaining weight. But there is a solution: eating foods low in sugar. Fresh fruits (a little), vegetables (a lot), nuts (very little) and protein such as lean meats (a lot) can do much to keep your blood-sugar levels stable and keep you from hitting the snack pantry.

By far a much healthier way to eat – satisfying your appetite with low-glycemic foods that keep you feeling full longer – can go a long way to helping you cut back on calories, while getting the good mix of fresh fruits and vegetables that you need to stay trim and healthy. *See the Appendix at the back of this book for a list of foods that are LOW on the glycemic index.*

Now, there are some exceptions. Pasta is on the list. However, it depends on what kind, how much you're eating and how you cook it. Pasta cooked until soft is higher on the GI. Avoid pasta for the initial month of making these changes. Then you can slowly incorporate al dente pasta (1 cup at a time) occasionally eaten on its own. I have highlighted in the Appendix which food low on the GI scale I recommend.

ACCORDING TO A STUDY IN THE JULY 2006 ARCHIVES OF INTERNAL MEDICINE, BOTH HIGH-PROTEIN AND LOW-GI DIETS INCREASE BODY-FAT LOSS. ACCORDING TO A STUDY IN THE ANNALS OF INTERNAL MEDICINE, "THE EFFECTS OF LOW CARBOHYDRATE VS. CONVENTIONAL WEIGHT LOSS DIETS IN SEVERELY OBESE ADULTS," A LOW-CARBOHYDRATE DIET (<30 GRAMS OF CARBOHYDRATES/DAY) HAD MORE FAVORABLE RESULTS THAN A CALORIE-RESTRICTIVE DIET (<30% OF CALORIES FROM FAT, A MORE CONVENTIONAL DIET), WHEN FOLLOWED UP ONE YEAR LATER.

This study suggests that the source of your calories matters. This means that is it better if your calories come from protein and good fats. **Avoid corn syrup, fructose, conventional honey and molasses.** These are refined and processed foods.

ACCORDING TO DR. DAVID LUDWIG OF CHILDREN'S HOSPITAL BOSTON, WE EAT 142 POUNDS OF SUGAR PER YEAR. THE AMERICAN ADULT FEMALE EATS 335 MORE CALORIES PER DAY THAN SHE DID 20 YEARS AGO. WE ARE 25 POUNDS HEAVIER THAN WE WERE 25 YEARS AGO.

If you need something sweet and fruit doesn't cut it, try a natural sweetener called stevia, and organic raw honey is all right in moderation.

Simple sugars (white sugar, refined sugar) enter the bloodstream quickly. The body releases insulin to keep blood-glucose levels from getting too high. Over time, the cells will burn out and stop responding to the signal and become insulin-resistant. Now, the body has to release more insulin because it cannot let blood-sugar levels get too high, creating too much insulin in the blood. Too much insulin for too long interferes with normal cell metabolism and increases inflammation. This will make it difficult to lose weight and cause a myriad of health problems.

ACCORDING TO THE JULY 2002 AMERICAN JOURNAL OF CLINICAL NUTRITION, LOW-GI FOODS CAN ASSIST IN WEIGHT CONTROL IN TWO WAYS: BY GIVING THE FEELING OF SATIETY (FEELING FULL) AND BY ALLOWING THE BODY TO BURN FAT INSTEAD OF CARBOHYDRATES.

RECENT STUDIES FROM THE HARVARD SCHOOL OF PUBLIC HEALTH INDICATE THAT TYPE 2 DIABETES AND CORONARY ARTERY DISEASE ARE STRONGLY RELATED TO THE GLYCEMIC INDEX OF THE OVERALL DIET. THE WORLD HEALTH ORGANIZATION (WHO) AND FOOD AND AGRI-CULTURE ORGANIZATION (FAO) ALSO RECOMMEND LOW-GI FOODS TO PREVENT CORONARY ARTERY DISEASE, DIABETES AND OBESITY.

The plan in this book will keep insulin levels in check, so you can lose weight without having to starve yourself. This explains why you may be so tired after you eat. Insulin resistance causes adrenal fatigue. When your adrenal glands don't work, you get very tired and then go for the sugar and the coffee to keep you awake. It's a vicious cycle. Can I just have a bite? No. It's not OK to just have a bite of something really bad for you, at least in the beginning. Your liver has a store of fuel called glycogen. Unless the store is depleted, your body will never go into the excess stored fat that has been there for so long. The liver will not go into its reserves if you have a big bite of chocolate cookie dough ice cream. That bite of ice cream will activate insulin. When insulin is present, the glycogen stores are inaccessible. A healthier, thinner person will use his or her body stores more efficiently. Once you become your ideal weight, you will be better able to process foods. Too much sugar also causes wrinkles – another reason to lay low on the carbs.

ACCORDING TO A STUDY IN THE 2007 BRITISH JOURNAL OF DERMA-
TOLOGY, HIGH-GLYCEMIC-INDEX FOODS (WHITE BREAD, PASTA AND
POTATOES) CAUSE ADVANCED GLYCATION PRODUCTS (AGES), WHICH
DAMAGE YOUR SKIN'S ELASTIN AND COLLAGEN. AGES CAN ALSO
DAMAGE YOUR BRAIN AND KIDNEYS. ANTIOXIDANTS HELP FIGHT
FREE RADICALS AND CAN PREVENT WRINKLES FROM OCCURRING.
CHECK OUT WWW.ITSNOTYOURFAULTYOUREFAT.COM FOR SOME
GREAT ANTIOXIDANTS SUCH AS CO-ENZYME Q10 TO HELP AVOID
THOSE WRINKLES. ALSO, EAT TOMATOES AND DARK-GREEN AND
ORANGE VEGETABLES FOR THEIR HIGH ANTIOXIDANT CONTENT.

GET AT LEAST 75 MILLIGRAMS OF VITAMIN C PER DAY. RESEARCH-
ERS HAVE REPORTED IN THE JOURNAL OF CLINICAL NUTRITION THAT
WOMEN 40 AND OVER WHO CONSUME ONE OR MORE ORANGES PER DAY
ARE LESS LIKELY TO GET WRINKLES BECAUSE VITAMIN C BOOSTS PRO-
DUCTION OF COLLAGEN, WHICH IS THE PROTEIN IN OUR SKIN THAT
KEEPS IT FIRM AND ELASTIC.

THE FOOD-HEALTH CONNECTION

In the past few decades, Americans have been getting fatter and
fatter, and sicker, too. Researchers studying the causes of so much
cancer and autoimmune diseases are focusing on our diets, because
what we eat has changed drastically over the last 25 years. We have
become a fast-food, processed-food and junk-food nation and we are
paying the price with our weight and our health.

CAPERS TO THE RESCUE!

RESEARCHERS FROM THE UNIVERSITY DE PALERMO IN ITALY HAVE
REPORTED THAT ADDING CAPERS TO YOUR RECIPES CAN – AND DOES
– HELP PREVENT HEART DISEASE AND CANCER. HOW? ACCORDING TO
THE STUDY, THESE TINY ANTIOXIDANTS HELPED PREVENT THE BUILDUP
OF DAMAGING DNA COMPOUNDS IN THE STOMACH.

The way we prepare our food may be making us sick as well. Recent research from Johns Hopkins University suggests that microwaves and plastic make for a deadly mix. That convenience may not be worth the health risk after all. Hormones in the plastic are able to leach into your food when you heat in plastic wrap or in microwave containers made from plastic. Use a plate or a glass dish to heat your food; it's much safer. Try using a toaster oven. Throw your microwave in the garbage! It kills your food and any nutrients in it. You may as well eat cardboard.

SUPPLEMENT FOR BETTER HEALTH

A multivitamin is a good idea for everyone and especially important when you are losing weight. The most important elements you need are the basic minerals that we should get from vegetables but are sometimes deficient because the soil they come from has been depleted of minerals. Calcium, Vitamin E, essential fatty acids and B-complex vitamins should also be a part of your daily ritual. These can be found in foods, but often we need much more than we could gain just from healthy eating.

DAILY VITAMIN RECOMMENDATIONS

1,200 MG CALCIUM
800 IU VITAMIN D
800 IU VITAMIN E
MULTIVITAMIN (INCLUDES ALL BS PLUS FOLIC ACID)
ESSENTIAL FATTY ACIDS (OMEGA-3S), FISH OILS
1 EXTRA ANTIOXIDANT (CO-ENZYME Q10)
PROBIOTIC

FOODS TO EAT APLENTY

WILD SALMON
GREEN LEAFY VEGETABLES
BERRIES
AVOCADOS
PINK GRAPEFRUIT
EGGS (YES, EGGS!)
RAW EGGS ARE FINE AS LONG AS THEY ARE ORGANIC.

HEALTHY CHICKENS LAY HEALTHY EGGS.

A little note on omega-3 fatty acids (fish oils): Everyone should be taking this supplement. Fish oils can boost your metabolism and burn up to 400 calories day by increasing the enzymes in your body that burn fat. They must contain EPA and DHA.

A STUDY IN THE JOURNAL OF THE AMERICAN COLLEGE OF CARDIOLOGY SUPPORTS THE BENEFITS OF OMEGA-3 FATTY ACIDS AS A NUTRITIONAL SUPPLEMENT, BUT ALSO AS A PREVENTION AND TREATMENT METHOD FOR PEOPLE WITH CARDIOVASCULAR DISEASE.

HEALTH BENEFITS OF TAKING FISH OILS

EPA AND DHA ARE POLYUNSATURATED OR ESSENTIAL FATTY ACIDS REFERRED TO AS "LONG-CHAIN" OMEGA-3 FATTY ACIDS, WHICH ARE FOUND IN HIGH CONCENTRATION LEVELS IN OILS FROM FATTY FISH LIKE TUNA AND SALMON AND VARIETIES OF SHELLFISH. THE LARGEST STUDY TO DATE OF THE CORRELATION BETWEEN OMEGA-3 FATTY ACIDS AND HEART DISEASE WAS THE GISSI PREVENTION STUDY (GRUPPO ITALIANO PER LO STUDIO DELLA SOPRAVVIVENZA NELL'INFARTO MIOCARDICO-PREVENZIONE). MORE THAN 2,800 ITALIAN HEART ATTACK SURVIVORS WERE GIVEN PURIFIED EPA/DHA IN CAPSULE FORM AND WERE ASKED TO TAKE ONE PER DAY FOR 3½ YEARS. EACH CAPSULE PROVIDED 850 MG OF EPA/DHA IN ROUGHLY EQUAL AMOUNTS. RESULTS SHOWED THAT DEATH FROM ANY CAUSE WAS REDUCED BY 20%, AND, INTERESTINGLY, SUDDEN DEATH (PRESUMABLY FROM A SECOND HEART ATTACK) FELL BY 45% COMPARED WITH A SIMILAR NUMBER OF PATIENTS NOT GIVEN THE

SUPPLEMENT. THE STUDY RESULTS POINT DIRECTLY TO EPA AND DHA AS THE AGENTS RESPONSIBLE FOR THE CARDIOVASCULAR HEALTH BENEFIT.

Check out **www.itsnotyourfaultyourefat.com** for the best-quality fish oils to add to your daily regimen.

4

◇◇◇◇◇◇◇◇◇◇◇◇◇◇◇◇◇

THOU SHALT GIVE THY BODY WHAT IT NEEDS (AND CRAVES)

Diets are often based on willpower. That's why, when you stray from a diet, the pounds creep back on. Most of us start a diet with good intentions and high hopes only to fall back into the same routines and give in to the same cravings that have gotten us into the plus-size section at our favorite clothing store. I can help – you need to break the cycle of eating for reasons other than hunger and then listen to what your body wants when it is truly hungry. Sounds simple enough, but let's take a look at what that means. What I am teaching you is not a diet, it is a lifestyle change, which will eventually become habit, so much so that you won't have to think too hard about it anymore; it will become second nature.

Imagine this, you are sitting at the computer, paying bills and you get that restless feeling, almost like an itch. Without even thinking, you head into the kitchen and start rummaging through the cabinets, looking for a quick fix for that craving. Salty or sweet? Hot or cold? You find some chocolate and head back to your spot, eating almost unconsciously as you continue the work. Is that a true craving? How about when you are ready for lunch and all you can think about is a big slice of pizza with pepperoni – nothing else will do? Or maybe it's a doughnut from that place down the street from your office, You know the feeling. It's more than hunger, it's that I-have-to-have-it-or-else kind of feeling that may or may not come in tandem with hunger.

So, are these cravings trying to tell you something? Does your body really need a slice of greasy pepperoni pizza or a doughnut? What about when it's not a specific thing – just that need for food that won't be satisfied until you've eaten? What's going on here and how can you make this time different – how, oh how, are you going to control your cravings and make your weight-loss goals a reality?

EMOTIONAL EATING

You know about this: Emotional eating is what so often trips us up when we are trying to diet. You're not hungry, but you can't stop thinking about your kids' Halloween candy that is sitting in a bucket on top of the fridge. Maybe the leftovers from that awesome restaurant are calling your name. You aren't really hungry; in fact, you aren't sure why you are drawn to eating. Let's take a look at what the emotional/physical connection is with food and why we so often feel powerless to our cravings.

We want food to satisfy our emotional needs. But it doesn't. That's the most important thing to remember here. We can make the choice to quell our anger, stress or sadness with a cookie or by facing those emotions in order to let them go and finding a new coping mechanism. When we are feeling down, our bodies are low on serotonin, a brain chemical that keeps our moods elevated and level. When the serotonin level drops, we are generally focused on getting it back up again and we feel a chocolate bar will do the job. But at what cost?

The cost of feeding our emotions is obesity. That's a fact. Our country has become obese because, unlike past generations, we turn to food for reasons other than hunger. Sugar can absolutely be addictive, and once we allow ourselves to rely on that quick sugar fix, we are in its grip until we make the decision to stop the vicious up/down cycle that comes with it.

If you find that you are eating at times of stress, boredom, frustration, anger, fear or shame, you are among the ranks of emotional eaters. Food is simply fuel for our bodies, but we live in a time (and a country) where the supply of food is generally abundant, as is the variety. Unlike our ancestors, we have become too pampered with food and have so many choices to satisfy every craving. Watch TV for an hour and you are bombarded with fast-food ads, snack-food ads, even an ad for a mini-cake that you can warm up in the oven to satisfy your chocolate craving and get that warm, cozy feeling that you got when your mom baked you cookies after school. It's no wonder so many of us have turned to food when what we really need is relief from stress or emotional distress.

What can you do if you're an emotional eater? Are you doomed to being overweight? There are better ways to satisfy your emotional needs; let's take a look at a few.

You are bored and restless, home alone and not sure what to do with your time, so you head to the kitchen for a quick pick-me-up. Stop and think before you feed that need. Instead of eating, try getting out of the house and taking a walk around the block. Give yourself some time to reset your mind and think about why you are eating.

You are anxious about work, worrying about whether there are layoffs coming to your department. You realize as you are walking toward the vending machine that you are en route to a big mistake. Again, stop! Take some deep breaths and turn around. When you get back to your desk, do a few stretches (as discreetly as possible) and then take several long, deep breaths. Increasing the amount of oxygen flowing through your body won't solve your work problems, but it will lift the general feeling of anxiety that has been creeping up on you all day.

Breaking the cycle of emotional eating can be very difficult, and failing to do so is the reason so many people find their weight creeping up again after losing it. If you can commit to feeding your body only when you are hungry, you will have won the battle against emotional eating. Here are some tips to stay focused on eliminating emotional eating:

- Eat only at the table – never on the phone, in front of the TV or computer.

- Portion out all your food onto a plate or into a bowl – don't eat anything right out of the original container unless it's already single-serving size.

- Change your habits – walk a different path to your office, avoiding the vending machine.

- Put up some encouraging notes to yourself or just tie a ribbon on the pantry door to remind yourself that you are only going to eat when you are truly hungry.

- Take steps to reduce your stress level before the cravings have a chance to hit – take up a hobby or start walking.

- Do not eat leftovers cold (heat your food).

Controlling emotional cravings is probably more than half the battle, and an issue that most diets don't address. It's great to know what to eat, but if you don't have the coping mechanisms to deal with your cravings, you are going to find yourself elbow-deep in the ice cream container! I remember watching my mom come home after work and eat from a box of crackers, eat some deli meat from the wrapper, eat a muffin, then take a spoon to the ice cream tub, all while standing up. Hmmm! I wonder if she had had a bad day. No wonder I ended up with some bad habits!

SOMETIMES IT'S OK TO SAY "YES"

You may not believe this, but every once in a while, it's actually OK to give in to your cravings, if you do it the right way. Most dietary experts agree that almost every weight-loss program works better if you don't feel deprived. Trying not to eat the food you love simply doesn't work for most people on a long-term basis, which can ultimately sabotage the best eating plan. You know the feeling. You're dying for pepperoni pizza, so you eat some grilled chicken. Then you have a salad. Then you try some rice cakes, and before you know it, you've downed twice the number calories of a small slice of your favorite pizza by trying to stop your craving for it.

The key to giving into those cravings is to change the way you think. Stop thinking like a fat person, who must down a whole pie (or even a whole piece). Instead, try thinking like a thin person. Your whole weight-loss process will be about not only stopping bad eating habits, but also replacing them with better ones. If you must have pizza, have your favorite kind, and have only one slice! It may sound impossible, but when you are eating well and exercising, you won't want to sabotage your efforts by regressing to your old habits.

A thin person will have pizza when she wants it, but she won't eat half a pizza and follow it up with an ice cream sundae. She will simply have a slice of pizza for dinner (probably with a salad) and be done with it. You can learn to do the same when cravings hit. Pick something you love, plan for it, and eat it in moderation. Don't grab snacks out of the fridge and eat while watching TV. Sit down and enjoy your snack – it will make it satisfying and not leave you craving more!

GIVING YOUR BODY THE VITAMINS AND MINERALS IT NEEDS

Once you recognize the vitamins and minerals in short supply in your body, the odds are that you will want to take some sort of supplement. While I'm all for taking quality, whole-food vitamins, I have to say that most of the vitamin supplements my patients bring to my office simply don't work. Why? Because they are synthetic varieties that simply don't contain enough of the vitamin and mineral needed to do much (if any) good. That's sad, considering how many people take these vitamins, thinking that they are doing something good for their bodies, when in reality they aren't doing much of anything to boost either their health or their weight-management routine.

WHY SYNTHETIC VITAMINS AREN'T GOOD FOR YOU

Most of the vitamins and supplements sold in stores aren't derived from whole foods (as they should be), but are made in a laboratory. Trying to find easy ways to both regulate vitamin supplements in the quest of making them safer and to mass produce supplements for easier use and expense, scientists have systematically found a way to make them ineffective. Most simply do not work.

The human body is designed to take in a variety of complementing enzymes, coenzymes and other vitamins and minerals through the food we eat; use what it needs; and excrete the rest. This is the way we get whole-food vitamins into our system.

When we synthesize vitamins for mass production, we only use a fraction of the actual vitamin. Whole vitamins are a combination of enzymes, trace elements and co-enzymes, all needed for the vitamin to work. Your body will treat any fractions of the vitamin as a foreign substance and will not be able to use it as intended. This can eventually cause biochemical imbalances and even toxic overload in some cases. As a matter of fact, research shows that taking synthetic vitamins regularly for a long period of time can cause both severe vitamin deficiencies and toxicity in most people. This can be really dangerous when dealing with some vitamins and minerals, since – without the right amounts – your heart, brain and other major organs can be at risk.

Let's look at a few examples:

1. When separated from its natural counterparts, Vitamin E is reported to lose 99% of its efficiency. In one study, the animals fed the synthesized Vitamin E supplement actually

died sooner than those not given any vitamins. That doesn't mean that your vitamin supplements are going to kill you – it does mean, however, they aren't helping you, either.

2. Synthesized B vitamins have shown no positive effect in some studies. As a matter of fact, many of the participants grew sicker taking the supplements, while those who were given a Vitamin B-rich diet grew stronger and healthier.

3. Taking ascorbic acid daily to help fight off colds and flu has been shown to reduce participants' white blood cells, thus compromising their immune systems.

Again and again, scientific research points to Mother Nature – and not synthetic supplements – as the answer to our health and diet woes. Nature has provided a perfect balance of what we need in our food and our environment. The key to a healthier life is to tap into those whole-food vitamins and minerals, leaving the synthetic ones alone.

Add to all of these dangers the fact that synthetic vitamins have very little nutritional value (maybe because they contain such a small amount of the vitamin itself), and one can't help but wonder what good taking your vitamins really does for you.

The fact remains that the average person does not get the right amount of vitamins and minerals from the foods he or she eats, and must supplement to keep healthy. But how can we be sure that the supplements we take are doing the job for which they are intended?

The first step is in buying only whole-food vitamins. Now, that doesn't mean that if the label says "all natural" and/or "organic" it's safe and effective. The odds are it isn't.

In order to be classified as "all natural," all a product has to do is contain some amount (no matter how minuscule) of an ingredient derived from nature. Since even the worst chemicals come from natural sources, virtually anything can be called natural by federal safety standards.

"Organic" is another term used lightly these days, since anything containing a carbon molecule can be called organic. Keep this in mind when seeking organic products: Even DDT has a carbon base and could be cited as an organic compound – scary, huh?

That said, there are a lot of all-natural and organic products that live up to their claims. It's your job as the consumer to make sure that what you buy indeed fits the bill. Some things to look for when purchasing vitamins supplements are:

- A laundry list of ingredients on the bottle. It should contain only a few.

- High dosages. Synthetic vitamins require taking more milligrams than whole-food vitamins and minerals

- Combination vitamins. It is virtually impossible to combine many vitamins naturally, so when you find a multivitamin that says it contains everything you need in a day, beware!

Did you know …

- *Thiamine HCL and thiamine mononitrate as B1 come from coal tar?*

- *D-alpha tocopherols as Vitamin E are processed and refined food oils?*

- *Vitamin C is made from refined corn sugars?*

- *DL-alpha tocopherols are made in a laboratory?*

SIDEBAR: NATURAL VS. SYNTHETIC

When looking at the ingredients on your vitamin bottle, you may be confused by the different names listed. That's why I have compiled this basic list of natural vs. synthetic ingredients, to help you make a better choice along the vitamin aisle.

This chart was extracted from *Going Back to the Basics of Human Health* by Mary Frost, a researcher and practitioner in the field of nutrition for more than 20 years:

NATURAL VITAMIN	SYNTHETIC VERSION
Vitamin A	Acetate, Retinal palmitate, Beta carotene
Vitamin B1	Thiamine HCL, Thiamine mononitrate
Vitamin B3	Niacin
Vitamin C	Ascorbic acid, Pycnogenols
Vitamin D	Irradiated ergosterol
Vitamin E	D-alpha tocopherol, DL-alpha tocopherol, D-alpha succinate
Vitamin K	K3 menadione

5

◇◇◇◇◇◇◇◇◇◇◇◇◇◇◇◇

THOU SHALT LEARN HOW TO SHOP FOR FOOD

Beginning a new weight-loss plan is a little bit like visiting a foreign country and you aren't quite sure if you are going to enjoy the trip. The atmosphere seems nice, but everything is so strange to you, it's hard to get your bearings. If you are feeling a bit wary about traveling to your healthier destination, take heart. Learning how to shop and how to read labels will be your travel guide and your pocket translator in a foreign land.

If you've tried to lose weight and failed, you may feel very apprehensive about trying again, and that is totally normal. The definition of success is not necessarily getting it right the first time, but rather to keep getting up when you fall. As the saying goes, you only have to get up one more time than you fall to be successful in anything, and weight loss is no exception.

CHANGE YOUR HABITS

Remember back in the first chapter we talked about our food histories? Well, I think it's time again for true confessions from me: When I was a kid I loved Chef Boyardee Beef Ravioli – loved it. Seriously, I ate pasta from a can – with meat, from a can. I then washed it down with a big glass of milk! It's actually shocking to write those words now as an adult, but as a kid it was my favorite food. My diet was full of processed and prepared foods and as I grew up, I continued to buy those types of foods for myself. The results, of course, were that I was overweight and had basically no idea how to feed myself in a healthy way. By the way, I do not recommend milk. Milk is one of the most common allergens, it creates inflammation, and if you have arthritis, it will give you a bad flare up! A very popular misconception is that we need to drink a lot of milk to get the calcium we need. This could not be further from the truth. Drinking milk does not ensure absorption of calcium, as you need approximately 12 other vitamins and minerals along with calcium in order for your body to access it.

Residents of the United States and Australia consume more dairy than those anywhere else in the world, yet have the highest fracture rates, whereas Asians and Africans consume little to no milk and their fracture rates are 50% to 70% lower than Americans'. Just consider this notion. We were raised to believe we should drink milk every day because that is what our parents were told. But if you were raised to believe the sky was green, you would grow up calling the sky green. We need to question everything we were told and not just accept all as fact.

WHY HARVARD RESEARCHERS DISCOURAGE MILK CONSUMPTION

ACCORDING TO A REPORT ISSUED BY THE HARVARD SCHOOL OF PUBLIC HEALTH IN 2005, DRINKING THREE GLASSES OF LOW-FAT MILK PER DAY, OR ITS EQUIVALENT DAIRY, ADDS MORE THAN 300 CALORIES A DAY TO YOUR OVERALL CALORIE INTAKE, WHICH CAN THWART YOUR DIETING EFFORTS. PLUS, THE STUDY CONTINUES, DRINKING SUCH LARGE AMOUNTS OF MILK CAN INCREASE YOUR RISK OF OVARIAN OR PROSTATE CANCER.

The only thing we need to drink is water. No store-bought fruit juices, no pop, no milk. Herbal teas are fine if you need a little flavor.

ACCORDING TO THE AMERICAN JOURNAL OF CLINICAL NUTRITION, WOMEN WHO DRANK MORE TEA PUT ON FEWER POUNDS OVER 14 YEARS THAN WOMEN WHO DIDN'T. THE PLANT-BASED ANTIOXIDANTS IN TEA, CALLED CATECHINS, WERE THOUGHT TO INCREASE THE BURNING OF FAT. GREEN AND WHITE TEAS CONTAIN THE HIGHEST AMOUNT OF CATECHINS.

To get the required calcium, eat foods from the following chart.

Calcium Content of Selected Vegan Foods

FOOD	AMOUNT	CALCIUM (mg)
Collard Greens, Cooked	1 cup	357
Turnip Greens, cooked	1 cup	249
Kale, cooked	1 cup	179
Okra, cooked	1 cup	172
Bok choy, cooked	1 cup	158
Mustard greens, cooked	1 cup	152
Tahini	2 tablespoons	128
Broccoli, cooked	1 cup	94
Almonds	1/4 cup	89

We will talk a little later about changing attitudes and exercising to help you lose weight, but at the most basic level, it's about changing your habits. You are where you are – whether it's 15 pounds or 150 pounds overweight. That can't be changed this instant. What you can do is start right now to make the big and small changes that will put you somewhere completely different in a few months. If you can make the changes I am suggesting to the way you shop for food, I promise you won't be getting a little heavier each year like you have been. You will be on your way to a healthy weight and lifestyle.

SHOP THE PERIMETER

Picture your local grocery store, the one where you shop the most. Think about what types of food line the perimeter of the store – the fresh ones, right? Grocery stores all have that in common – the freshest food is kept around the perimeter to make restocking easier. Produce needs to be put out and maintained daily and those fresh fruits and veggies come to your store already chilled. The same thing is true for meats, poultry and fish: they are constantly being brought in and stocked.

The vast middle of the store does have redeeming qualities and you will still need staples like extra-virgin olive oil. The freezer section won't be off-limits either, but you won't be spending much time in the wasteland of prepared foods and sugary snacks. Your new destination is all about freshness and nutrients – no more Twinkies, no more chips, and definitely no more Chef Boyardee! Stick to the outer edges of the grocery store and your cart will be full of healthy and fresh foods rather than the processed poison that is lurking in the middle.

BUY LOCAL

Your town probably has a farmer's market, especially through the spring and summer months when produce is abundant. You will never find a fresher tomato or a tastier pepper than one you buy right from the grower – even the eggs are likely to be free-range and organic. We have grown so accustomed to buying whatever type of produce is available at our neighborhood grocery or the superstore where we also buy our shampoo and laundry detergent. What we all need to learn is that buying organic, in-season and locally grown produce is better for us, better for our local economy, and better for the environment.

You would actually be shocked if you knew what was in your food, including pesticides and other chemicals. That quick rinse in the sink before you make your salad is definitely not enough to get those toxins off your produce. The only way to avoid ingesting them is to purchase vegetables and fruits that were organically grown without any chemical enhancement.

When you are starting to fill your diet with fresh produce and meats, it may take a while for your palate to adjust to the changes in taste. After all, fresh pineapple can be very sweet, but nothing is as sweet as a sugar-frosted donut. A lifetime of making poor food choices has trained your palate to enjoy super-sweet, super-salty and greasy foods rather than the natural tastes you were meant to crave. It will take some time to get used to the flavors of fresh fruits, but choosing the freshest, in-season ones will make that transition much easier. A fresh-picked peach is miles away from one that has taken a long journey to get to your grocery store's shelves.

If the taste alone weren't enough to sell you on the idea of buying locally grown produce, the impact it has both on your area farmers and the environment should push you over the edge. You may even be able to find a farm co-op or share program where you can purchase a portion of the harvest. Developing a taste for fresh produce will be much easier if you are eating the best and freshest available.

READING LABELS

Now that you've got your map to this new land of healthy eating, you need a good translator. After all, when you were overweight, you didn't have to worry about what you were buying; you simply purchased what you liked and would taste good or give you a little boost in the moment. For your new destination, you will need to learn to read food labels – the ingredients, the nutritional breakdown and the serving sizes. Learning to read a nutritional label will be invaluable in making healthier choices and in losing weight.

INGREDIENTS

Of course, all packaged foods have a list of its ingredients, but some are hard to find and others are impossible to pronounce. Many foods that claim to be "all-natural" or "low-fat" will have an ingredient list a mile long that includes several if not all words that you won't be able to pronounce (and shouldn't be eating). A good guide when looking at the ingredients is that a long list is generally a bad thing. If what you are eating has an ingredient list a mile long, it's most likely full of artificial flavors, colors and fillers. Hydrogenated oils, monosodium glutamate and high fructose corn syrup are among the biggest offenders when it comes to packaged foods. Also, choose foods low on the glycemic index to prevent spikes in your blood sugar.

Another thing to keep in mind is that the ingredients are listed from the largest quantity ingredient to the smallest. So, if the second ingredient in your snack is salt, you can bet it is chock-full of it; if your boxed soup has salt as the second to last ingredient, you are probably OK. You will also find that many foods claiming to be low-fat are packed with sugar, and many claiming to be all-natural contain large amounts of corn syrup or hydrogenated oils – both of which are natural but unhealthy! It may seem confusing at first, but the more you read and, more important, compare food labels, the better you will become at making informed choices. And, carefully choosing what you are going to eat, taking all factors into consideration, is a great way to get started on losing weight and keeping it off.

SIDEBAR: INGREDIENTS TO WATCH OUT FOR

If there is one thing I hope you have learned so far, it is that you can enjoy eating healthy fresh foods. Unfortunately, it isn't always easy to know whether the foodstuffs you're buying are indeed good for you. Learning to read the labels will help, but honestly, what should you be looking for? Here are some of the biggest health and weight culprits around. Check the label to see if your favorite foods contain high levels of any of these ingredients, and if they do, look for a substitute:

1. **High fructose corn syrup (HFCS)** - Found in virtually every food on store shelves, high fructose corn syrup may be the No. 1 obesity contributor of modern times. Found in our juices, cereals, sauces, ketchup, barbecue sauces, hamburger buns, and more other products than I can list

here, it may seem impossible to live without it, especially if you are looking to buy prepackaged food items rather than fresh. Too much of it can – and will – deteriorate your health and make you fat, so be sure to limit products containing it as much as possible. (We eat 63 pounds of HFCS per year!) HFCS is found in soda pop. You must eliminate soda pop. If you stop drinking pop and store-bought fruit juice you will lose weight just from making this one change.

ONE CAN OF POP IS 150 CALORIES X 365 DAYS PER YEAR DIVIDED BY 3,500 CALORIES PER POUND = A 15½-POUND WEIGHT GAIN PER YEAR.

---

2. **Enriched and bleached flour** - Just because a product claims to be made from wheat or whole grains doesn't mean that it is made from 100% whole grain products. Actually, finding 100% whole grain products isn't easy, since most manufacturers combine enriched wheat with whole wheat to save money.

To be sure that you are getting the whole-grain product you want, look for the words "enriched" or "bleached" on the label. They're a tip-off that the product isn't 100% whole grain in origin. Why is it so important to avoid enriched and bleached products? Basically, the enriching and bleaching process strips the nutrients and the fiber from the wheat, which turns these healthy whole grains into nothing more than an empty-calorie carbohydrate. Why can the Italians eat all the pasta they want and not get fat? They use a hard wheat called durum wheat, which is not stripped of nutrients and digests much more slowly. Anyone want to go to Rome? By the way, contrary to popular belief, I do not recommend whole grains or any grains for that matter. Avoid rice even (brown rice), wheat, gluten, rye, mullet, barley, quinoa, buckwheat, cereals and oatmeal! Many people cannot digest these foods and it wreaks havoc on their systems. *Micromiracles* by Dr. Ellen Cutler explains this very well.

3. **Trans fats** - "Trans fats" has been a real buzzword lately and for good reason: They are horrible for you! Some countries even ban trans fats in food. They have been directly linked to high cholesterol and heart disease, yet many food manufacturers continue to insist that without them the taste of our food would suffer. Still, many states and cities are beginning to ban the use of trans fats in restaurants and processed foods sold within their boundaries. Still, be sure to look carefully for "trans fats" on every food label and avoid them like the plague. Your heart will thank you for it.

4. **Foods with 10 ingredients or more** - As I said earlier, the more ingredients in a product, the less pure it seems to be. Here's a good rule of thumb: If a food product contains more than 10 unpronounceable ingredients, leave it on the store shelf. It isn't good for you and it certainly isn't good for your waistline.

5. **Artificial colorings** - You may have heard about allergies to artificial colorings from your child's classroom, but have you ever considered what this simple ingredient is doing to your health and weight? Linked to such serious illnesses as cancer, tumors, and allergic reactions, artificial colorings should be avoided. FYI: red dye or food color is the worst offender.

6. **Saturated fats** - A definite contributor to obesity, saturated fats aren't all bad. They do contain some good stuff, too, but must be eaten in moderation to ensure that they won't sabotage your weight-loss plans.

7. **High sugars** - Sugar sure has gotten a bad reputation in recent years. While a little should go a long way, most of us have overindulged in this sweet treat for so long we have no idea what moderation means. The basic facts are these: Refined, white sugar has no nutrients and is basically empty calories and carbohydrates. So stay away from it.

8. **High sodium** - People totally underestimate the use of sodium (or salt) these days. Foods you wouldn't ever think had sodium in them – like milk and pop – often have more than the daily recommended allowance for a single serving. This can be detrimental to your diet, since salt makes you retain water and can make you look puffy and swollen. Plus, too much sodium in your diet can and will affect your heart by increasing your blood pressure. When deciding whether or not a certain food contains too much salt, remember this important guideline: You should take in only 2 grams, or 2,000 milligrams, of sodium per day. This may sound like a lot, but once you start reading those food labels, you'll soon realize that it isn't. Sodium intake adds up quickly, so be watchful.

9. **MSG (monosodium glutamate)** - MSG is a salt of glutamic acid, an amino acid used as a flavor enhancer. It has raised a lot of concern over the years. Excessive MSG consumption can cause some mild to severe symptoms in some people,

including headaches, fatigue, nausea and possibly even cancer.

10. **Sodium nitrate** - This is a preservative found in processed meats such as hot dogs and deli meats, salami, bologna and ham. It is used to preserve color. Without it, the meat you buy wouldn't look nearly as good. It is best to avoid all processed meats, as they contain chemicals that have been shown to cause cancer in animals.

These ingredients may have a direct effect on your diet and they can have an effect on how much weight you lose by making your body less able to metabolize the food and calories you take in, absorb the proper nutrients, and keep working at peak capacity – all things that are necessary in order to maintain a healthy weight.

Foods to Avoid (recap)

HIGH-FRUCTOSE CORN SYRUP
FRUCTOSE
SUCROSE
SOY (DEPRESSES YOUR THYROID AND SLOWS METABOLISM)
ARTIFICIAL SWEETENERS
STORE-BOUGHT FRUIT JUICE
MILK
ENERGY DRINKS
SODA POP
WHITE SUGAR/WHITE FLOUR
SATURATED FAT
COFFEE

NUTRITIONAL BREAKDOWN

Those numbers on the side of the package have important meaning for your new weight-loss plan. The information contained in that little grid of abbreviations and numbers is an essential tool for weight loss. The typical food label lists the calories, fat content and breakdown, cholesterol, sodium, carbohydrates and protein. Beyond those basics, many vitamins and minerals may be included, but they are generally to sell you on a product and, although the information is valuable, it isn't essential for your weight loss. Also, your diet will be full of fresh fruits and vegetables that will give you plenty of nutrients. What is good to know is:

1 gram of fat = 9 calories

1 gram of protein = 4 calories

1 gram of carbohydrates = 4 calories

The fats on the nutrition label will be broken down into:

- *Total fat*

- *Saturated fats (bad)*

- *Unsaturated fats (good)*

- *Trans fats (very bad)*

Saturated fats are generally those from animal products, dairy and a few tropical oils. Unsaturated fats (which are much healthier) are those derived from plant sources.

When looking at a nutritional label, you must remember that the percentages they give are based on a daily value not on a serving size. If your snack contains 50% of the daily value of fat, that does not mean it is 50% fat: it means that the snack you are about to eat contains half of the fat you should eat in an entire day. The label will give you all the information you need to understand your food; you just need to take the time to read it carefully.

SERVING SIZE

The final piece of the puzzle when it comes to reading food labels is serving size. Let's face it, we are living in the land of the gigantic portion and have pretty much forgotten what a healthy food portion even looks like. All the nutritional information, the calories, the fat, the protein, is based on the serving size suggested on the label. One serving may be one small crumb, so watch the labels.

When you are portioning out your food, it's a good idea to measure your serving sizes just to get the hang of it. You don't have to get a food scale and attach the measuring cups to your belt loop, but you do have to familiarize yourself with what an appropriate portion looks like. Once you know, you will be able to retire the measuring cups, secure in the knowledge that you are, in fact, eating a single serving! A good general rule of thumb is that one serving is about the size of a fist.

Shopping for food is a basic part of your weight-loss plan, but if you skip the basics, you won't achieve your goals and you will struggle with your weight loss from the very beginning. Making a plan for the store, never shopping when you are hungry or upset, and sticking to the outside edges will put you on the right path to a thinner and healthier future!

SIDEBAR: EATING OUT WITHOUT SABOTAGING YOUR DIET

It's your birthday and your spouse wants to take you out for a romantic dinner. Should you go? While you would love to spend some alone time out having a scrumptious dinner for two, you can't help but wonder if one evening of indulgence is worth the 75 minutes of cardio it'll require to take those calories back off of your hips and thighs.

Let me reassure you of one thing: Getting those extra pounds off and keeping them off doesn't require giving up every romantic dinner, or even staying out of your favorite restaurant forever. Otherwise, I would have ditched my new eating plan eons ago. If you haven't guessed it by now, let me tell you my little secret: *I love to eat and I love to eat food prepared by someone else!* I'll bet you do, too. So, instead of ditching a favorite pastime and a rare evening out, let's look at ways we can both have our cake and eat it too – well, at least some of it!

Eating out at a restaurant occasionally (keyword here: occasionally) doesn't have to mean moving up a dress size. It does mean learning a few tricks that will let you enjoy your favorite foods without the guilt or the need to unbutton your pants afterward – and you thought untucking your shirt was new fashion trend! It's just a way to hide our bulging bellies.

Ready to learn how to eat out smarter? Good! I'm ready to show you. OK, so let's start as soon as you walk in the door of your favorite restaurant and are seated. Do you immediately reach for the breadbasket and order a cocktail? Now, that could be a problem. Ask the server to hold off on the bread. This will keep you from mindlessly munching as you sit chatting, waiting to be served your meal. If you must eat something, ask for your salad or veggies first. And, when it comes to that pre-dinner cocktail, forget the beer, heavy liquor and carbonated drinks. They will just make you eat more. One glass of red wine is usually OK or some vodka with soda and squeeze of lemon or lime. No more than one drink!

Once you have been seated and gotten your drink, it's time to pick up that menu and decide on your main course. As we have already discussed, when ordering appetizers, always opt for a healthier, leaner choice, or if you must have those specialty items, split the order with the rest of your party.

When ordering your meal, keep these important tips in mind:

- Be sure to order several steamed vegetables instead of rice, potatoes, fries, pastas and other grains. Whenever you can, substitute mushrooms for pasta or rice.

EAT MUSHROOMS TO WARD OFF ILLNESS AND BOOST WEIGHT-LOSS TOTALS. ACCORDING TO RESEARCHERS AT TUFTS UNIVERSITY, EATING WHITE BUTTON MUSHROOMS HAS BEEN SHOWN TO BOOST THE IMMUNE SYSTEM'S ABILITY TO PRODUCE KILLER CELLS, WHICH CAN WARD OFF VIRUSES AND TUMORS. PLUS, SUBSTITUTING ONE CUP OF MUSHROOMS FOR ONE CUP OF RICE OR PASTA CAN HELP YOU LOSE WEIGHT, TOO, SINCE YOU'LL SAVE 200 CALORIES AT EACH MEAL.

- Order good protein like chicken, shrimp, fish or lean beef.

- Ask how your food will be prepared: Will it be sautéed in butter – which is OK – olive oil (fine) or vegetable oils (no good)?

- Avoid creamy sauces and soups.

ACCORDING TO AMERICAN INSTITUTE OF CANCER RESEARCH IN WASHINGTON, REPLACING BUTTER, CHEESE OR CREAM WITH MASHED AVOCADO NOT ONLY HELPS TO REDUCE CALORIES BUT ALSO INCREASES THE HEALTHY MUFA (MONOUNSATURATED FATTY ACIDS) INTAKE.

- Ask for any sauces on the side, but keep in mind that the server will likely give you twice the amount you would have received on your plate, so spoon out a tablespoon or so and have the rest taken away.

Once your food arrives, you will want to be sure to leave some on your plate – actually about one-third. According to a study presented at the American Diabetes Association's annual meeting a few years ago, more than 40% of people underestimate how much they eat – especially when eating out.

We've been taught that if it is on our plate, we should eat it. Wait! There's that old advice again drilled into us by our mothers. You don't have to eat everything on your plate. As a matter of fact, you shouldn't. Most restaurants serve way more food than we need to feel satisfied, so feel free to push your plate away before polishing off all of the food. Here's a good rule to follow: If you eat a fistful of three veggies and one protein, you've given your body what it needs for that meal. Eat more and you are overindulging.

The Chinese eat until their stomachs are 80% full. If you can't tell when that is, try eating more slowly and, when you're satisfied, stop. When you feel uncomfortable or "stuffed," you have gone overboard. Start paying attention to how you feel after you have eaten and you will slowly develop a sense for this.

Want to see what got you into that larger size skirt? Just take a look at your plate the next time you dine out. The odds are there are a lot more than four fistfuls of good food on it. Don't get suckered into believing you must eat it all – you don't!

Now, here's the rule I hate the most. Never take any food home from a restaurant. I personally have a hard time with this one for several reasons:

1. I've paid for that food.

2. I want those leftovers.

As hard as it may be to decline that little Styrofoam box, do it. Taking your leftovers home will only entice you to eat them, and gain weight.

OK, you've made it through the appetizers and the main course, now your server is returning with – oh no – the dessert cart! What's a gal on a diet to do? Have a hot cup of herbal tea and skip dessert or just leave the restaurant!

At first you may worry that eating out will sabotage your weight-loss plans. Here's hoping you now see that enjoying dinner out with your partner or friends is just fine, as long as you follow a few simple rules.

ACCORDING TO THE AUGUST 12 ISSUE OF THE JOURNAL OF THE AMERICAN MEDICAL ASSOCIATION, FOLLOWING A MEDITERRANEAN DIET AND ENGAGING IN HIGHER LEVELS OF EXERCISE WERE ASSOCI-ATED WITH A LOWER RISK OF ALZHEIMER'S DISEASE. THIS DIET IS HIGH IN FRUITS, VEGETABLES, LEGUMES, FISH AND OLIVE OIL AS THE MAIN SOURCE OF MONOUNSATURATED FAT.

6

◇◇◇◇◇◇◇◇◇◇◇◇◇

THOU SHALT MOVE THY BODY!

We are well on our way to setting up a healthy lifestyle that will help you shed pounds and feel great, but we haven't yet discussed one of the most important factors in weight loss: EXERCISE! What's that? Did I hear a groan? Maybe you are already imagining squeezing your plus-size body into some Spandex outfit and heading to the fitness center for Barbie-style aerobics? Maybe you are envisioning long days spent on a treadmill or stationery bike?

ACCORDING TO JOHN JAKICIC, PHD, FACSM, AND THE CHAIR COMMITTEE ON OBESITY PREVENTION AND TREATMENT FOR THE AMERICAN COLLEGE OF SPORTS MEDICINE, THE EVIDENCE IS CLEAR WHEN IT COMES TO THE LINK BETWEEN EXERCISE AND WEIGHT LOSS/WEIGHT MANAGEMENT. "PHYSICAL ACTIVITY IS AN IMPORTANT COMPONENT FOR INITIAL WEIGHT LOSS," HE SAYS. IN A STUDY HE RELEASED IN 2008, JAKICIC SHOWED THAT HIGH LEVELS OF EXERCISE (275 MINUTES ABOVE BASELINE LEVELS) CONTRIBUTED TO THE PARTICIPANTS' GREATEST WEIGHT LOSS OVER A TWO-YEAR PERIOD.

Well, you do have to exercise if you truly want to be healthy, but I am going to tell you the secret: You might just enjoy it! There is no magic exercise that will make you thin, no set of abdominals that will give you a six-pack, no expensive exercise DVD set that will make you model-thin in a month. Here's the secret to exercise:

1. Pick something you enjoy.

2. Do it (almost) every day.

3. Push yourself to improve.

You are probably thinking that it can't be that simple, right? If you've spent any time watching infomercials you might think that you need some special equipment or videos or a gym membership to get into shape, but the truth is, you don't. Of course, if what you love is going to the gym for aerobics classes, then, by all means that is what you should do. But, if you just like to walk and listen to music, put your headphones on and head out the door. Stick with it and you will lose weight and be healthy!

If you are one of those who despise exercise and cringe at the thought of going to the gym, just go outside and walk at any pace. Build up to 30 to 60 minutes per day. Make it a priority.

CARDIOVASCULAR EXERCISE

We hear a lot of hype about the type of exercise, but let's take a look at what it actually means. Cardiovascular exercise is physical activity that raises our heart rates for an extended period of time. That might sound like a bad idea at first, but the heart is a muscle and needs to be used and worked to function at its best. When the heart is healthy, it can work more efficiently, pumping more blood with fewer contractions in a resting state; when it is unhealthy, it has to work much harder to circulate the same amount of blood through the body.

During aerobic or cardiovascular exercise, the heart increases its speed and gains strength so that it can work better when you aren't exercising. Like any other muscle, the heart needs to be used to get stronger, and the stronger your heart is, the healthier you are.

The American Heart Association recommends that healthy adults get a minimum of 30 minutes of moderately strenuous exercise most days of the week. The benefits of exercise are well known and well documented, but for our purposes, what you need to know is that regular exercise will help you drop pounds! It's that simple – exercise, eat healthy and lose weight! Your moods will improve, your health will improve and you will get thinner by making regular exercise a part of your life.

Here are some ideas for a cardio workout to get you started:

- WALK! Probably the simplest exercise you can do and one of the most effective. Just put your sneakers on and get out there.

- Run: You may not be ready to run just yet, but if you start out with walking and add some running to your exercise routine, you will be surprised how quickly you will improve.

- Fitness classes: If you join your local health club (or are already a non-active member) you will find tons of classes, from kickboxing to salsa dancing, all of which will give you a great workout and some camaraderie.

- Swimming: This is a great option for people who have a lot of weight to lose or who have joint problems. Get in the water for some lap swimming – it's a wonderful cardio workout with little or no impact.

- Cycling or spinning: Whether you head out on your bike or to the gym for a spinning (stationery bike) class, cycling works the large muscle groups as well as the heart.

- Organized sports: Fast-paced sports like soccer or basketball are a great workout and offer the benefit of being on a team with other people. They also often don't feel like exercise!

- Go paint the town red and DANCE the night away (belly dancing is really fun).

STRENGTH TRAINING

Just as there are conflicting theories about how much and what type of cardiovascular exercise is the best at helping you lose weight, there is much discussion about strength training, especially for women.

Strength training can improve your posture, make you look taller and leaner as you are losing weight and improve your ability to burn fat. As you increase your muscle mass, you become a more efficient calorie burner and your metabolism gets a boost from the amount of muscle you have on your body. Women absolutely need a higher percentage of fat in their bodies than men do (otherwise, how would we have any curves?), but most women have too much fat. Beyond obesity, a high body fat percentage can have health risks and cause hormonal imbalances. A healthy body fat percentage is between 20% and 30% for women, with anything over 33% considered obese.

The good news is that you can improve your body fat percentage by losing weight and increasing muscle. Your cardiovascular exercise will keep your heart in good shape and burn calories, while the strength training will build lean muscle and improve strength and flexibility. Some great strength training methods are:

- Circuit training: Your fitness center probably has a pre-set exercise routine on the weight machines that will be a great place to start a strength exercise plan.

- Free weights: Simple exercises with handheld weights are great for building muscle and can be easily done at home.

- Resistance training: Using bands or an exercise ball, these types of exercises are simple and you don't need gym or a class to do them.

Other exercises that increase flexibility and strength, such as yoga and Pilates, are wonderful for improving your body shape and for relaxation.

PICK SOMETHING YOU LOVE

All right, maybe you can't even imagine loving exercise, but if you truly dislike the type of exercise you choose, you will have an even harder time sticking with a program than if you even sort of like it. There are so many ways to exercise, there is bound to be one you enjoy

---

STUDY PROVES THAT A LITTLE EXERCISE IS JUST AS GOOD AS A LOT!

THE NATIONAL HEART, LUNG AND BLOOD INSTITUTE (NHLBI) HAS BEEN STUDYING THE EFFECTS OF EXERCISE ON WOMEN FOR A LONG TIME, AND RELEASED A STUDY A FEW YEARS AGO THAT SHOWED MODERATE PHYSICAL ACTIVITY DID JUST AS MUCH FOR A WOMAN'S ABILITY TO LOSE WEIGHT AS AN INTENSE WORKOUT DID. ACCORDING TO THE STUDY, WHICH TRACKED THE WEIGHT-LOSS RESULTS OF 201 OVERWEIGHT WOMEN BETWEEN THE AGES OF 21-45, THOSE WHO PARTICIPATED IN STRENUOUS PHYSICAL ACTIVITY FOR AT LEAST 45 MINUTES PER DAY AND WOMEN WHO SIMPLY TOOK A BRISK WALK FOR THE SAME AMOUNT OF TIME LOST ROUGHLY THE SAME AMOUNT OF WEIGHT, WITH BOTH GROUPS KEEPING IT OFF FOR A SUSTAINED AMOUNT OF TIME.

THE FACT REMAINS THAT PARTICIPATING IN SOME ACTIVITY – ANY ACTIVITY – FOR AT LEAST FIVE HOURS A WEEK (OR ABOUT 45 MINUTES PER DAY) WILL GIVE YOU THE SAME RESULTS AS HITTING THE GYM FOR THE SAME AMOUNT OF TIME.

MAKE TIME FOR EXERCISE

We know we should exercise, don't we? But there is always something else to do, whether it's the laundry, driving the kids somewhere, grocery shopping or even catching the latest episode of our favorite shows. We let life get in the way of exercise, right?

I will go out on a limb here and say that if your best friend or your husband or your kids needed something right now, you would drop everything and do it for them, am I right? Or at least, am I close? Now, what if you treated yourself like you were just as important as all those people? Well, guess what? You are that important. As you begin to adopt this new healthy lifestyle and you are losing weight and feeling better, you will start to see that not only is it OK to put yourself first (at least sometimes), it's essential to your success. If you keep putting exercise on the back burner, you will find yourself continuing to gain weight year after year after year. Once you have made the switch to putting exercise on your schedule, you may even find it hard to remember when it wasn't. It will become as natural as brushing your teeth or answering your e-mail.

So, I challenge you to write your exercise plan into your calendar each week; make a plan and stick to it. Consider that spinning class or that time with the treadmill to be an appointment as unbreakable as a job interview or check-up with your dentist. You are important and your exercise time is necessary for your health and your weight loss! At the beginning of each week, make a note of when and how you will exercise each day and keep those promises to yourself. The results will be worth the work, believe me.

You may not be able to devote hours of each and every day to exercise, but you can manage 30 minutes almost every day; everyone can! Don't watch TV at night; don't surf the Internet; get out and get moving.

PUSH YOURSELF

Once you have committed to an exercise routine, continue to set goals for yourself. You are not at the gym or on the track to just put in your 30 minutes; you are there to make real changes in your life, your health and your appearance. If you are walking a 20-minute mile this week, try for a 19-minute mile next week. If you are jogging for 10 minutes and walking for 20, try to make it half jogging and half walking. Stepping up your exercise plan will keep your weight loss steady and pay off big time in your overall health. Don't think of exercise as a punishment for being overweight; accept it as part of your new healthy life. Some of the other benefits of exercise, beyond weight loss are:

- Increased energy and stamina

- Better mental focus

- Increased sex drive

- Better posture

- Reduced risks of disease

- Improved moods and reduction of stress

Regular exercise will really improve your life as a whole. And, beyond the scheduled exercise you are committing to, you can incorporate more activity into your daily life and your family's life. Make a family walk after dinner your new tradition – it will keep you off the couch and foster closeness and communication with your family. Take the stairs whenever possible and park farther away from your office or the mall. Find ways to put activity into your life!

7

◇◇◇◇◇◇◇◇◇◇◇◇◇◇◇◇◇◇◇

THOU SHALT DRINK ENOUGH (WATER, THAT IS)

You may find this hard to believe, but I once had a patient who admitted to me that the only water she consumed was the ice that she put in her soda! Can you imagine how dehydrated her body was? You've heard it all before; our bodies are made up of mostly water and that every cell in them contains water. But what does that really mean for us? Most people are walking around already dehydrated. If you feel thirst, that's your body's signal to tell you to drink; at that point, you are already behind the eight ball with hydration. Before you ever begin to feel thirsty, your health is at risk if your body doesn't have the proper amount of hydration. Your immune system begins to break down at just slight dehydration, which can make you susceptible to a number of potentially dangerous diseases.

The Hydration Report, an important study conducted in 1999 throughout 100 workplaces, found that at just 2 percent dehydration, most people's work begins to suffer; 4% dehydration resulted in some real side effects including lethargy, bad temperament, stress and even nausea.

Our bodies crave water, just water. Not flavored water, not diet soda (gasp!) or regular soda, not coffee or tea or iced tea or store-bought fruit juice – just water. We need it to survive and we need plenty of it to really thrive. Deprived of water, the human body can last only a short time before kidney and liver function are affected and symptoms of shock begin to set in. The more water you drink, the better able your liver and kidneys are to flush toxins from your body. Water increases your organs' abilities to process waste, keeping every system in your body working at peak capacity.

The liver may be the most hard-working organ in the body when it comes to detoxification. If it does not get enough hydration, the liver can go into overload, which stresses your entire body and leaves many toxins from the food you eat and the environment remaining. This can cause some serious health effects down the line.

You may think that your kidneys' only job is to flush excess fats and substances from the body. That's only part of their story. Your kidneys actually purify your bloodstream, and if they are working too hard because of a lack of water, they can't keep your bloodstream pure. This can cause a variety of problems including:

- Dry, flaky skin

- Headaches

- Insomnia

- Lack of concentration

- Susceptibility to infection

- Anxiety

- Depression

This may all sound a bit daunting, especially if you find yourself suffering with some of these symptoms. But, there is plenty of good news. First, all of these symptoms can be alleviated simply by taking in the proper amount of water each day – approximately eight glasses per day for most people. And no, the water in iced tea, lemonade, pop or coffee does not count as part of the water intake.

Second, it is important to understand that most of us suffer from lower levels of dehydration, causing fatigue, dry skin, constipation and water retention. By drinking more water, you can easily stop further damage to all of your bodily systems. Also, the more water you drink, the less you will eat.

A WATER-WISE DIET REALLY WORKS

A STUDY BY DR. BRENDA DAVY, ASSOCIATE PROFESSOR AT VIRGINIA TECH SHOWED THAT SUBJECTS WHO DRANK TWO GLASSES OF WATER 20-30 MINUTES BEFORE A MEAL LOST MORE WEIGHT, MORE QUICKLY THAN THOSE WHO DID NOT. A FOLLOW-UP STUDY FOUND THAT SUBJECTS WHO FOLLOWED THIS PROGRAM CONSUMED AN AVERAGE OF 75 FEWER CALORIES PER MEAL, WHICH WAS WHAT ACTUALLY CAUSED THE WEIGHT LOSS.

THE DANGERS LURKING IN YOUR WATER

Now you know the importance of drinking more water, but should you be concerned about the water you are drinking? Unfortunately, not all water is created equal. There are some real dangers lurking in your tap water that you should be concerned about. Heavy metals may be in the water you drink, cook with and even shower with. Over time, they can build up in your system and cause heavy metal toxicity, which has been linked to conditions such as Alzheimer's disease and even cancer.

So, what are some of the biggest dangers in today's water supplies? Here are a few to watch out for:

CHLORINE

Chlorine is one of the most popular chemicals used to purify drinking water in the Western world. Chlorine is essentially bleach. It destroys the normal intestinal flora that helps you digest. It is not uncommon for chronic skin conditions like acne, psoriasis, seborrhea and eczema to clear up or to be significantly improved by switching to unchlorinated drinking water and supplementing the diet with lactobacillus acidophilus and bifidus. It is also a carcinogen (known to cause cancer).

FLUORIDE

Believe it or not, it is illegal to add fluoride to the water in many countries (including Germany, France and Spain). Why? Because these countries have discovered that the chemical can cause some very serious health concerns including Down's syndrome, multiple birth defects, and severe allergies. In addition, it is believed that fluoride toxicity interferes with the metabolism of calcium, magnesium, manganese and Vitamin C – all of them important components to good health and weight loss.

ALUMINUM

The most bountiful metal on earth, aluminum sulphate is a common water treatment chemical used to keep our water supply safe. Unfortunately, some research studies have linked high levels of aluminum with Alzheimer's disease.

CALCIUM

Can the water you drink actually make you fatter? It can, if it has been stripped of its important minerals, thus making it into a refined food product. While the other chemicals listed above were considered dangerous when found in water, calcium is actually needed to help your body. The problem is that, while we add so many chemicals to our drinking water to keep it safe, we take out this much-needed mineral, which in turn strips the water of important minerals, which can make it no better for us than a refined food product – something that is no good to our waistlines.

HOW MUCH WATER DO YOU REALLY NEED?

The guidelines vary from source to source and depend on factors such as age and the level of physical activity in which you engage. If you are running three miles a day, you will certainly be losing more fluids than a person your age who is sitting at a desk all day. The eight, eight-ounce glasses a day rule is a general guide for water consumption. But that is just a start, if you factor in exercise and the amount of caffeine you consume per day. Caffeine acts as a diuretic, taking water out of the body. Each caffeinated beverage you consume, including coffee, depletes your body of a cup of water, so you would need to drink two glasses of water to counteract the diuretic effects of the caffeine.

When you are exercising, you must stay hydrated. Drinking water before, during and after a workout will ensure that you have the stamina and coordination to complete your workout. Don't ruin the benefits of exercise by depriving your body of water and putting it under unnecessary stress.

NO coffee allowed. Coffee contains caffeine (no decaf either), which can wreak havoc on your adrenal glands and create an imbalance in your hormones and affect your blood sugar. You can also lose minerals such as calcium, magnesium, sodium, chloride and potassium.

ACCORDING TO THE OFFICE OF DIETARY SUPPLEMENTS, NATIONAL INSTITUTE OF HEALTH, HIGH AMOUNTS OF CAFFEINE IN THE BODY CAN INCREASE EXCRETION AND REDUCE ABSORPTION OF CALCIUM. THIS IS SUPPORTED BY STUDIES PUBLISHED IN THE INTERNATIONAL JOURNAL OF MOLECULAR SCIENCES IN MAY 2008, WHICH SHOWED CAFFEINE CONSUMPTION WAS A RISK FOR OSTEOPOROSIS. IN THE EXPERIMENT, RATS EXPOSED TO DIETARY WATER CONTAINING HIGH AMOUNTS OF CAFFEINE LATER EXHIBITED BONE MINERAL DENSITY LOSS.

One way to evaluate your hydration is to look at your urine. Yes, I did just tell you to look in the toilet. Urine should be pale in color, almost colorless, with the exception of your first urine of the day, which is generally a little darker as a result of your body storing it overnight. Dark urine is a sign that something is wrong and you need to get hydrated. Just as with persistent thirst, if you have consistently dark urine that doesn't seem to respond to hydration, it's time to contact your health care provider.

Rise and Shine: Your body loses a lot of water throughout the night, so be sure to drink at least one eight-ounce glass as soon as you get up, either warm or room temperature. Never put ice in your water, it will shock the stomach. Never drink water cold unless you are overheated.

During Your Commute: Be sure to sip on a bottle of water during your commute to keep from getting dehydrated on your way to work.

Midmorning Water Break: Take a midmorning water break (around 11 a.m.) to both curb your need for a sugary snack and to give your body the water it needs to keep going (and lose weight).

Pre-Lunch Water Snack: One of the best ways to keep from overindulging at lunchtime is to drink eight ounces of water 20-30 minutes before you head out for your midday meal.

Midafternoon Pick-Me-Up: The best way to keep a clear head for the end-of-the-day chores is to down eight ounces of water around 2 p.m.

End-of-Workday Treat: End your workday with another glass of water in order to ensure that the commute home won't be dehydrating.

Before-Dinner Drink: Cocktails before dinner may help to calm your nerves after a stressful day at work, but they sure can add to your waistline. Opt for a soothing warm glass of water about a half-hour before dinnertime instead.

Before-Bed Ritual: Relax with a glass of warm water two hours or so before bed to give your body the proper hydration to get through the night. Be careful, though, not to drink it too close to bedtime, lest you risk having to get up during the night to use the bathroom.

CHOOSING THE BEST WATER

Who knew there were so many ways to prepare drinking water? Take a look around: there's bottled water; spring water; filtered water; tap water (gasp!); energy water, and more. When did water get so complicated?

The important thing to remember when choosing your water is that just because it is expensive or sports a fancy label, that doesn't mean it's the best water out there.

Consider this: Research conducted by the U.S. Environmental Studies Institute shows that 24 out of 37 bottled water brands studies did not comply with official standards. That's a lot of bad water being sold out there. Now, that's scary!

Sometimes the best way to ensure that your water is clean and safe for consumption is to get a quality filter for your faucet. Filtered water comes in a lot of varieties, with each stripping away different chemicals and toxins. A carbon filter, for example, may help your water to taste (and smell) better, but it will do little to take out those heavy metals and bacteria you're worried about. A reverse osmosis filter is best for getting bacteria, pesticides, heavy metals and other toxic chemicals out of your water. The problem is it also takes out important trace minerals. So be sure whatever filter you choose leaves these important minerals in.

If you are worried about your skin absorbing toxins through the water you shower in, bathe in, and inhale through steam, then a whole-house filter may be your best bet. A cheaper fix is a shower filter, which is a simple attachment to your showerhead available at any local hardware store.

You can practice these simple water-purifying techniques:

- Never drink tap water, or well water unless it is filtered.

- Drink good-quality bottled spring water, or filtered water from the tap is acceptable (do a water analysis if you're not sure about the quality of your water).

- Buy a filter for your tap.

- Get a special attachment for your showerhead. (Available at hardware stores)

- Get a water filter (Brita is a good one) if you do not have a filter on your tap

WHAT ABOUT SODA?

Soda is criminal, if you ask me. Yes, I think it is that bad for you! I've already shared with you my bout with kidney stones that was a result of my over-consumption of diet soda, but there is more. The sugar in regular soda can add thousands of calories to your diet every week even if you have only a glass or two a day. And, just as with many other foods in our super-size culture, a bottle of soda that you get from a vending machine or convenience store may be two or three servings rather than one. Pop is poison!

STUDIES CONDUCTED AT RUTGERS UNIVERSITY IN 2007 SHOWED THAT BEVERAGES MADE WITH HIGH FRUCTOSE CORN SYRUP HAVE HIGH LEVELS OF REACTIVE CARBONYLS – A FREE RADICAL LINKED TO TISSUE DAMAGE, THE DEVELOPMENT OF DIABETES AND DIABETES COMPLICATIONS. PEOPLE WITH HIGH CONSUMPTION OF SODA DRINKS ARE LESS LIKELY TO HAVE SUFFICIENT INTAKES OF VITAMIN A, CALCIUM, OR MAGNESIUM. THE LOSS OF THESE VITAL MINERALS IS ATTRIBUTED TO HIGH SUGAR CONTENT, WHICH DEPLETES MAGNESIUM, AND TO THE HIGH LEVELS OF PHOSPHORIC ACID IN SODAS THAT COMBINE WITH CALCIUM AND MAGNESIUM IN THE DIGESTIVE TRACT.

So if you are drinking one 20-ounce bottle of soda per day, you are contributing 240 empty calories to your daily intake every single day. With those calories, you are getting no nutrients, no protein and no fiber, and you aren't hydrating your body either. An ice-cold soda on a hot day may taste good, but it doesn't do anything for your health. Just eliminating that one soda will result in a savings of 7,200 calories in just one month! That is a lot of calories wasted on a sugary drink.

ACCORDING TO THE 1994-1996 AND 1998 CONTINUING SURVEY OF FOOD INTAKES OF INDIVIDUALS (CSFII), WHICH CONSISTED OF SAMPLE INDIVIDUALS IN 50 STATES, THE AVERAGE DAILY INTAKE OF SOFT DRINKS MORE THAN DOUBLED FROM 5 FLUID OUNCES IN 1977/78 TO 12 FLUID OUNCES IN 1994/98. DATA ANALYZED SHOWED THAT AMONG PRE-SCHOOL-AGE CHILDREN, SCHOOL-AGE CHILDREN AND ADOLESCENTS, 50%, 64%, AND 82%, RESPECTIVELY, CONSUMED SOFT DRINKS IN THE TWO-DAY DIETARY SURVEY. THE INCREASE IN SOFT DRINK CONSUMP-TION SHOWED A DECREASE IN THE CONSUMPTION OF MILK, FRUIT JUICE, AND THE NUTRIENTS CONCENTRATED IN THESE HEALTHIER BEVERAGES.

Diet soda is full of artificial sweeteners and flavors and, as mentioned before, is a poor substitute for the sugary snacks you might be craving. Not to mention the fact that it is poison. Ten percent of the aspartame you consume becomes methanol, or wood alcohol. One can of diet soda has 16 milligrams of methanol. The EPA has determined that people should not consume more than 8 milligrams of this dangerous substance a day. Even at cold temperatures, methanol can also break down into formaldehyde, which may disrupt cellular function and DNA (J. Seminars in Cancer Biology 1998; 8:255). According to Dr. Joseph Mercola in *Sweet Deception*, artificial sweeteners are a major contributor to obesity and cellular breakdown. So make sure you don't crack open that pop after you let it sit it the car all day (that's even worse). Regular consumption of diet soda is actually linked to weight gain rather than weight loss, as well as a host of other health issues and sensitivities.

DIET FOODS WITH ARTIFICIAL SWEETENERS WILL MAKE YOU GAIN WEIGHT

THE RESULTS OF A STUDY BY PURDUE UNIVERSITY WERE RELEASED IN FEBRUARY 2008 IN THE JOURNAL BEHAVIORAL NEUROSCIENCE. THE STUDY REPORTED THAT RATS ON DIETS CONTAINING THE ARTIFICIAL SWEETENER SACCHARIN GAINED MORE WEIGHT COMPARED WITH RATS THAT WERE GIVEN REGULAR SUGARY FOOD. THE RATS APPEARED TO EXPERIENCE A PHYSIOLOGICAL CONNECTION BETWEEN SWEET TASTES AND CALORIES, WHICH DROVE THEM TO OVEREAT.

A very common problem is headaches. I have had patients whose headaches completely resolved after removing diet pop. Studies on aspartame and other artificial sweeteners show that these sugar substitutes are actually harmful and should be avoided. Another ingredient in diet soda, phosphorus, actually steals calcium from your bones. That's a quick way to get osteoporosis!

THE USE OF ARTIFICIAL SWEETENERS SUCH AS ASPARTAME, SACCHARIN AND ACESULFAME-K, AMONG A FEW, HAVE BEEN ASSUMED TO BE THE HEALTHIER OPTION COMPARED WITH USING SUGAR, AS IN THE CASE OF REGULAR VS. DIET SOFT DRINKS. HOWEVER, DIET SODAS HAVE BEEN FOUND TO ACTUALLY CONTRIBUTE TO WEIGHT GAIN. RESEARCHERS AT THE HEALTH SCIENCE CENTER IN THE UNIVERSITY OF TEXAS LOOKED AT EIGHT YEARS OF DATA FROM 1,550 PEOPLE AGES 25 TO 64. THEY WERE SURPRISED TO FIND THAT PARTICIPANTS WHO WERE DRINKING ONLY DIET SOFT DRINKS HAD HIGHER RISK OF OBESITY THAN THOSE WHO WERE DRINKING REGULAR SOFT DRINKS. THERE WAS A 41% INCREASE IN THE RISK OF BEING OVERWEIGHT FOR EVERY CAN OR BOTTLE OF DIET SODA A PERSON CONSUMES DAILY.

64 OUNCES EVERY DAY?

At the minimum, you should be striving to get your eight glasses of water every day. If you are the type of person who has a cup of coffee in the morning and then a soda with dinner and nothing in between, this will be quite an adjustment. We all tend to drink a little more when the weather is hot or when we are exercising or sweating from yard work, but it's just as important to drink water when you are sitting at your desk all day. Getting used to life without soda, whether diet or regular, isn't easy for some people. Maybe that soda at midmorning gives you a little sugar rush and some energy to last until lunch. You should replace that soda with water and a healthy snack that will boost your energy level and provide some nutrition instead of the empty calories you found in that soda can.

Here are some ideas of how to get your water consumption up:

- Carry a water bottle with you. Get used to it; with your new, healthy lifestyle, water will be your best friend. Drinking from a 20-ounce or bigger bottle will encourage you to drink more throughout the day.

- Add a little lemon. Lemons are very good for the digestion and they add some flavor to your water, which is especially helpful for people who are used to sweet drinks.

- Drink as soon as you wake up – a glass of warm or room-temperature water is a great way to start the day. I recommend a tall glass of warm water when you first get up in the morning to rehydrate and relax the stomach to prepare it for breakfast.

- Head off your snack cravings with water and you may just be able to forgo that snack after you feel full with water.

Once you get your water consumption up to a good level, you will start to feel more rested, your skin will have a glow, and you will feel much less bloated. It seems counterintuitive, but when you deprive your body of water, it retains whatever water it has, actually making you carry excess water weight. Once you have flushed out your system, so to speak, you won't have to retain that water and you will lose that extra weight. You will notice the most difference at the beginning of your water regimen, but you will keep that light, refreshed feeling as long as you stay hydrated.

Take a pass on fancy coffee drinks. If you must have coffee, opt for black, no more than one cup a day. Coffee does contain some antioxidants, but once you add chocolate, cream, and who knows what else to get your long-named drink at the coffee shop, you might as well be having a slice of cake. Ideally, no coffee at all.

Alcohol is a depressant and it depletes the body of water. For the most part, you will want to avoid cocktails, regular beer and wine coolers. If you really want a drink, opt for red wine with its powerful antioxidants, but be careful. Drinking alcohol often goes hand in hand with overeating, and you don't want to accidentally ruin all your hard work by munching on peanuts at the bar!

A NOTE OF CAUTION

When I was a kid, my mom always encouraged us to drink a lot of water with meals. While the advice on the water may have been good, the timing was way off. Remember we talked earlier about the digestive enzymes that are hard at work in your system when you are eating? Well, those can't really do their jobs if they are diluted with water. That slows the digestion by making it more difficult to break down your food. The longer the food is in your digestive tract, the worse it is for your health. Therefore, just drink enough water needed so you don't choke while eating.

Avoid drinking water that has been heated in plastic, such as the water you left in a plastic bottle in your warm car. Toxins in the plastic bottles leach into the water when the plastic is heated. These toxins are thought to contribute to the growth of cancer cells. Use glass containers whenever possible or choose one of the many nonplastic but still reusable options available for water bottles. You will help the environment while you are keeping harmful materials out of your system.

Remember, water is the best, healthiest and most efficient form of hydration you can give your body. Stay hydrated and your body will perform better, feel better and look better!

8

◇◇◇◇◇◇◇◇◇◇◇◇◇◇◇◇◇

THOU SHALT STOP FALLING FOR ALL OF THOSE DIET PROMISES AND MYTHS

What if I told you that the secret to weight loss was bacon – that's right good old- fashioned salty, smoked pork bacon? Just have a slice of bacon with every meal – with eggs and toast for breakfast, crumbled on a salad at lunch, and wrapped around a steak at dinner. It doesn't matter what else you eat, the grease in the bacon will actually coat your digestive system and allow all the fats and sugars in the food you eat to simply pass through your body. The good stuff, the protein and complex carbs along with the nutrients you need every day, will be able to break through the grease barrier and enter your system. You should lose about 10 pounds per week with the bacon diet and won't even have to exercise!

Are you on to me yet? Have you figured out that my "perfect diet" is a scam? I am sure you saw right through my bacon diet, but you have probably believed the hype of other diets and made yourself crazy trying to follow their rules so that you, too, could lose weight without exercise or changing your habits. If you have, take heart. You are not alone; the diet industry is a billion-dollar money-making machine. If even some of those fad diets worked, the number of obese Americans would not be rising each year, it would be dropping quickly as everyone would follow the plan that works.

The sometimes hard-to-hear truth is that there is no magic pill, no powder, no potion, no secret mixture of food that will make you thin. Most of us gained weight through a combination of genetics and habits, and we got this fat over time, so it will take time to get the weight off. Anyone who promises instant results is definitely trying to sell you something, and a lot of it! The nitty-gritty of healthy eating is that you will need to eat better; what you eat has to be more nutritious. You will also have to increase your activity level. If you follow that plan and stick with it, you will have great results – it may not be overnight, but we all know that slow and steady usually wins the race.

Many people are able to stick to a very restrictive diet plan for a short time and lose even a substantial amount of weight, but they cannot maintain that loss because they go off the diet. They haven't made the fundamental changes necessary for real and lasting weight loss; they have simply been in diet overdrive to lose as much as they can as quickly as they can.

Fad diets are popular because even though we all know that we really can't lose 20 pounds in a week, we would love to believe that we could. Whether you have 25, 50, 100 pounds or more to lose, the road ahead looks scary and long and you aren't sure you are ready to run this race again. You are thinking that you don't know whether you can make the changes you need. And, why should you make those changes when the latest diet craze is just telling you to eat bacon at every meal – that sounds easier!

THE MAJOR OFFENDERS

Some diets just keep popping up in a new form or with a new twist, but they share some commonalities. Here is a sampling of the major categories of fad diets:

EXCLUSION DIETS

The Atkins diet falls into this category, because it touts the elimination of an entire food group, identifying carbs as the enemy in the battle against weight and promising quick results with a protein-heavy diet. Many people did lose weight using this type of diet, which only helps to support the myth that it's a great way to take off pounds. We all know people who did lose weight when the Atkins was all the rage, but have they kept it off? If they have, then they are definitely in the minority, because most people who lose weight with a fad diet find that the minute they resume a normal diet, the weight comes back fast and furious. They may even find that they are heavier than before they ever started the diet!

One of my patients loved the idea of a quick-fix diet and chose the high-protein, no carbohydrate route. She was initially thrilled with the results, because she was eating eggs, bacon, hamburgers and cheese and still losing weight. What was not to like? After a month or so on the program, her weight loss slowed to almost a standstill and she came to me complaining of dizziness and confusion. It seems that a month of nearly binging on high-fat meats and cheeses had taken its toll.

We need a variety of food for good health and weight maintenance. The fiber and nutrients in fresh produce is without equal, and these need to be a part of a healthy diet. Developers of fad diets that blame a single food group need to go back to health class and learn their lessons about a balanced diet!

THE MAGIC PILL

Supplements, diet pills and diet shakes seem to be the fool's gold of the diet world. We would all like to believe that simply taking a pill will help us lose weight, but most don't help and some are downright dangerous, especially for people with health conditions like high blood pressure and diabetes.

Many diet pills combine appetite suppressants, which inhibit your natural hunger, with caffeine, which replaces the energy lost when you eat less. They also often have a diuretic component that rids the body of excess water weight (which we know should be done by staying hydrated). This combination sets you up to lack real energy because you have stifled your natural hunger, which is your body telling you it needs fuel. You will still feel like you have energy, thanks to the caffeine, but now you are feeling lethargic because the buzz has worn off and you are dehydrated.

Prescription medications and diet pills can be tempting because they seem to promise a quick weight-loss solution. Many have proven to be unsafe. Taking a prescription pill for weight loss only confuses your body. If weight loss were only physical it would be so much simpler, but true and lasting weight loss encompasses your whole life and must be a lifestyle change.

Only by answering your body's need for food with healthy and nutritious choices can you really find the energy you need and lose weight. The better-quality food you put in, the more energy you will have.

Protein bars, meal replacements and energy bars are all the rage. If you are only eating meal "replacements" you are almost certain to bounce back to your original weight (or higher) when you return to regular eating. I would avoid all these. Avoid fad diets, as they are calorie-restrictive, making them very difficult to maintain for any length of time and they often send the body into famine-mode and makes it hold onto fat rather than shedding it. Again, a balanced diet, full of real, flavorful and healthy food is the best way to lose weight and to keep it off.

Our culture is one of instant messaging, microwave dinners and downloadable music, so of course we are vulnerable to the promises of a quick fix when it comes to weight loss. It can be hard to stay the course and stick with a weight-loss plan, but the payoff in the long run will be more than worth the effort you put into it.

9

THOU SHALT LEARN TO RELAX

You've had a bad day at work; layoffs are rampant at your job and you think you might be next. You finally head out, 40 minutes later than usual, only to find that someone has scratched the door of your brand-new car! The traffic is terrible and your boyfriend or husband calls your cell while you are sitting on the exit ramp to tell you he is heading out with some friends, hope you don't mind. How do you react? If you are thinking that you need some chocolate (or ice cream or chips) then you are like many, many people who use food to ease their stress.

Certainly, the feeling of satisfaction that comfort food provides, or the quick sugar rush of chocolate, will help you feel better in the short run. You may even experience a sense of calm the moment you start having your snack; you have trained yourself to use food for a purpose other than fuel for your body. You comfort yourself with it and use it to relieve stress. You are in good company, believe me. Millions of overweight people react in the same way when they feel stress taking over their bodies and minds, and that is how we ended up overweight. The conscious mind knows that eating a big bowl of ice cream isn't a good idea, but the subconscious wants that fix, that instant calm that we have trained ourselves to receive from eating.

STRESS AND WEIGHT

So, does stress cause weight gain? Yes. The effect of stress on our lives is so enormous and far-reaching that it does have implications on our weight. For those of us who are genetically prone to weight gain and obesity, dealing with stress is an important issue to handle if we want to get in control of our weight. A hormone that packs on the pounds for many of us when we are under consistent stress may be in play; it's called cortisol, and it is secreted in our bodies when we are stressed. Long- term stress and excessive cortisol have an effect on our weight gain. Therefore, managing your stress levels is important.

Beyond the biological sources of weight gain, the more likely culprits are our coping mechanisms. If we are conditioned to self-soothe with food, then any type of stress is going to send us running to the freezer for that ice cream. Only when we change the way we cope with stress can we expect to start losing weight.

NEW STUDY LINKS EMOTIONS TO OVEREATING

IF THE STRESS IN YOUR LIFE SENDS YOU STRAIGHT FOR THE SNACK CUPBOARD, THAN YOU MAY BE ONE OF THE MILLIONS OF PEOPLE A NEW STUDY CONDUCTED BY THE MAYO CLINIC WARNS COULD BE AT RISK FOR EMOTIONAL-EATING OBESITY. ACCORDING TO THE STUDY, RELEASED IN AUGUST 2009 BY THE MAYO CLINIC'S WOMEN'S HEALTH-SOURCE, "THE CONNECTION BETWEEN STRESS AND EATING LIKELY HAS ROOTS IN BRAIN CHEMISTRY." THIS IS CAUSED, SAYS THE REPORT, BY THE FIGHT-OR-FLIGHT REACTION THE BODY ENACTS TO DEAL WITH STRESS.

"FACED WITH REAL DANGER, THE FIGHT-OR-FLIGHT REACTION KICKS IN AND SUPPRESSES APPETITE TEMPORARILY," READS A PRESS RELEASE

DISTRIBUTED BY THE RESEARCH TEAM CONDUCTING THE STUDY. "BUT WHEN FACED WITH PERSISTENT STRESS, MANY PEOPLE TURN TO HIGH FAT, HIGH-CALORIE FOODS FOR COMFORT." THIS CHEMICALLY INDUCED COPING MECHANISM DOES OF COURSE MAKE THOSE TURNING TO FOOD AS A STRESS RELIEF MORE PRONE TO BE OVERWEIGHT.

THE KEY TO OVERRIDING WHAT YOUR BRAIN IS TELLING YOU TO DO (EAT) WHEN STRESSED, URGES THE REPORT, IS TO LEARN TO RECOGNIZE TRUE HUNGER; LOOK ELSEWHERE FOR COMFORT; IDENTIFY FOOD TRIGGERS; PRACTICE MINDFUL EATING; AND FIND OTHER WAYS TO REDUCE YOUR STRESS.

Of course, if your stress is getting to be more than you can handle, it may be time to seek some help. Constant stress, such as caring for a sick family member, divorce, loss of a job, or the death of a loved one can send you spiraling out of control. It can lead to fatigue, depression and even isolation. If you have gained weight due to depression, you may feel ashamed and become unable to go out and be around friends and family, never mind strangers. If you are feeling completely overwhelmed with the degree of stress in your life, you should reach out to your health-care provider, therapist, or a trusted friend or family member. There is help for depression and anxiety and you don't have to do it alone.

Dealing with ongoing stress can cause headaches, fatigue and loss of interest in activities you used to enjoy, all of which can contribute to weight gain. You may be thinking of taking a walk, but a headache and tiredness head you off at the pass. Instead you reach for some candy or cookies and enjoy the sugar high for as long as it will last. Stress can be a vicious cycle; once you feel stressed, you eat and gain weight. Then, the weight causes more stress and makes it harder for you to make the changes necessary for losing weight. Only by changing your coping mechanisms and learning to handle stress and relax will you be able to pursue a healthy lifestyle and lose weight. Also, stress affects women differently than men. Does your husband or partner ever say to you, "Don't worry about it!" only to make you even more upset? Well, according to a new study, women and men gain weight differently.

IN THE AMERICAN JOURNAL OF EPIDEMIOLOGY, RESEARCHERS FROM HARVARD'S SCHOOL OF PUBLIC HEALTH FOUND THAT WOMEN GAINED WEIGHT DUE TO A WIDER VARIETY OF STRESSORS THAN THOSE THAT AFFECT MEN. THE STUDY FOLLOWED 1,355 MEN AND WOMEN OVER NINE YEARS AND CONCLUDED THAT MEN GAINED WEIGHT WITH ONLY TWO STRESSORS, BOTH BEING RELATED TO WORK. WOMEN GAINED WEIGHT DUE TO POOR FINANCES, TENSE JOBS, STRAINED FAMILY RELA- TIONSHIPS, AND LIMITED LIFE CIRCUMSTANCES. ALSO, THOSE WOMEN WHO WEIGHED THE MOST AT THE BEGINNING OF THE STUDY GAINED SIGNIFICANTLY MORE WEIGHT THAN THE LIGHTER COUNTERPARTS.

MAKE CHANGES FOR GOOD

Relying on food for stress relief will always end in failure. You can't just eliminate your coping mechanism and expect to feel OK the next time you are stressed out; you need to replace it with a healthy alternative. Here are some simple ways to calm your nerves and avoid the pantry:

- Take a walk. Just once around the block may be enough to settle your emotions and work out whatever is stressing you. This can be especially helpful right after a hard day at work.

- Listen to music. Retreat to a private spot in your home and put on some relaxing music (headphones are especially good for blocking out other noise). Really listen to the music and let your mind settle.

- Call a friend. Sometimes, you need a sympathetic ear, and calling a friend is a great way to blow off steam. Just make sure you are there to return the favor sometime when she needs it, too!

- Drink. No, not a cocktail, just a tall glass of warm or room-temperature water.

- Clean. Yes, I said clean. Sometimes if you are angry or frustrated, a little bit of housecleaning can be just the thing to get out whatever is bugging you, and you get a clean house out of the deal.

- Read. Pick up a book or a magazine and get in your comfy chair and read for a few minutes.

- Meditate. There are many different techniques. If you picture a bunch of monks chanting as the only form of meditation, try getting Wayne Dyer's "Getting into the Gap" CD; it is a good start and not weird at all.

- Weigh yourself daily. This may not be a stress reliever; however, I believe it is important. You often wonder how people gain 10 pounds, then 20 pounds then 30 pounds then 40 pounds then 100 pounds. At some point they give up, and never weigh themselves again. If you weigh yourself daily it will be less likely the numbers will climb and more likely you will do something about it. Don't worry if it's plus or minus a few, it takes time for your body to adapt. Also, if you're using weights, you may gain a little initially as you burn fat and gain muscle. It's OK. Don't be a slave to the scale. It doesn't help you.

Probably the best way you can reduce the effects of stress on your life (because, let's face it, we can't really get stress out of our lives for good) is EXERCISE! Regular exercise helps balance our emotions, gives us energy, and changes the actual way our brains work, giving us a boost of serotonin that a candy bar can't compete with! Although you may not be able to hit the gym every time you feel stressed out, having a good, regular exercise regimen will help you manage the stress you feel on a daily basis, even when you are not exercising at that exact time. It's like a savings bank of calm and you are training your brain to react differently to stress every time you exercise.

RELAXATION TECHNIQUES

Yoga and other relaxation exercises have been used for centuries to improve flexibility and to calm a restless spirit. The slow movements of the yoga poses help your muscles to stretch and contract, releasing powerful hormones in the muscles that help cultivate a feeling of relaxation. But, you don't have to enroll in yoga to benefit from some simple stretches and breathing exercises that will help you handle the stress of everyday life.

- Just breathe: Sounds simple enough, doesn't it? You would be surprised how often you hold your breath when you are stressed. Taking shallow breaths is nearly as bad; you can oxygenate your whole body with just a few deep, slow, purposeful breaths.

- Calgon, take me away: Picture yourself somewhere soothing: a beach, a cozy spot in your home, in the woods. Find your special place and stay there for a minute or longer. You will find that your heart rate will slow and your body will relax.

• Unclench: That includes your teeth, your fists, even your butt cheeks! Stress translates itself into a physical reaction when we unknowingly tighten our muscles. Taking a moment to purposefully relax each muscle in your body, starting at the head and working down to the toes, can release frustrations and stress.

AN EASTERN APPROACH

You may not be familiar with traditional Chinese medicine because our culture seems to be all about the pharmaceutical and not about the natural, almost mystical philosophies that abound in this ancient practice. In Chinese medicine, it's all about the Qi (pronounced and often spelled "chi" in English), which is the spiritual energy or life force that runs through us. When our Qi is blocked, we cannot handle stress and illnesses occur more frequently. Acupuncture is a way to open up the channels in our bodies and allow the Qi to flow more freely.

Having needles stuck into your skin may not sound like your idea of a good cure for stress, but people seek out the help of acupuncturists and hypnotists to help them handle stress and weight loss. I have recommended acupuncture and hypnosis for my patients when I felt either could help them, and a reputable acupuncturist can work wonders for someone struggling with stress and weight gain. Also, chiropractic can help by keeping your nerves functioning properly and your joints moving well. Massage therapy can also assist in relaxing your muscles.

Whatever method you choose to reduce and relieve your stress, it can only help you on your journey to lasting weight loss. Many of us have turned to food in every difficult situation, so it can be a hard habit to break. Once you find a good replacement for food when you are stressed, you will be able to finally break that cycle. It might even be a good idea to make a list of all the ways you can handle your stress and post it on the fridge. That should be a good deterrent when you slip into your old ways. Foods that help decrease stress contain Vitamin B6, such as nuts, and B12, such as salmon.

10

THOU SHALT ADJUST
YOUR ATTITUDE

Many people who have never dealt with a weight problem are under the wrong impression about fat people. They believe that fat people are lazy and don't want to do anything about their weight, or that they just simply don't care. Nothing could be further from the truth, and if you are like most overweight people, you spend a good part of your day berating yourself for all the mistakes you have made that day and for how you look. People who struggle with weight also struggle with a very negative internal dialogue.

I first realized that I was really overweight when I was about 10 years old. I think I was in the fourth or fifth grade and I was taking Ukrainian dance lessons. I was so excited to try on the beautiful flowered skirt that we were all going to wear for a performance. It came with an ornate belt that was supposed to wrap around the waist several times to finish off the outfit. When it was my turn to get fitted, I was mortified. The belt went around my middle only once when it easily went around the other girls several times. I could feel my face get red, and I knew right then and there that I was different, and didn't like it. I was already fighting a battle with my weight and I knew that I was losing. Even though I couldn't put it into words at the time, my self-esteem took a big hit that day.

If you stood naked in front of a mirror right now, how would you feel? What would be going through your mind as you looked at your body? I am sure you wouldn't have anything nice to say to yourself at all, would you? Well, that defeatist attitude has something to do with your weight problem, and you have to change it if you want to lose weight – that's a fact! The things we tell ourselves are incredibly powerful, and if you are constantly reminding yourself of your weight and your failures at losing weight, you will be your own worst enemy throughout this process and probably will not succeed at achieving weight loss. It's that important.

YOUR THOUGHTS REALLY CAN MAKE YOU FAT

ACCORDING TO NANDO PELUSI AND MITCHELL ROBIN, CLINICAL PSYCHOLOGISTS IN NEW YORK CITY, THE MESSAGES WE SEND OURSELVES MAY BE SABOTAGING OUR WEIGHT-LOSS EFFORTS. THOUGHTS SUCH AS "I MUST BE THIN" CREATE A SENSE OF DESPERATION, WHICH WILL ULTIMATELY UNDERMINE YOUR DIETING EFFORTS, WHILE THE THOUGHT THAT YOU NEED COMFORT FROM THE FOOD YOU EAT WILL ONLY SEND YOU RUNNING TOWARD THE WORST STUFF IN THE PANTRY. IN ADDITION, TELLING YOURSELF THAT YOU CAN'T STICK TO A DIET WILL SUCCEED ONLY IN FRUSTRATING YOU AND TAKING AWAY YOUR MOTIVATION. SO BE CAREFUL WHAT MESSAGES YOU SEND YOURSELF WHILE TRYING TO LOSE WEIGHT – IT COULD MAKE THE DIFFERENCE BETWEEN SUCCESS AND FAILURE.

BE YOUR OWN BEST FRIEND

Think now about your best friend. She is complaining about her weight – how much she hates her stomach, her thighs, and she really hates her butt. What would you say to her? Would you agree or would you offer to work out with her or maybe just empathize with how she is feeling? Would you tell her it's her own fault for eating so many loaded tacos for lunch every day or would you understand her frustration and try to make her feel better? If you are a good friend, you will take her side every time and encourage her to do better. You wouldn't treat a friend the way you treat yourself, would you?

Well, maybe it's time to start treating yourself like a friend. Every time you want to tell yourself you are fat, you can't lose weight, or that you are going to fail, concentrate instead on telling yourself something positive. You chose a good breakfast; you stayed on the treadmill 10 minutes longer today; you went for a walk after work instead of snacking on chips and dip. Find something positive to say to yourself, even if it feels funny at first. Concentrate on who you are. You are not your weight – you are a friend, a wife, a mother, a sister, an aunt. All the good things that you are for all the people you care about are way more important than your weight. It's time to stop beating yourself up. A great technique to help you deal with your feelings and clear your mind is found at www.releasetechnique.com. This technique has helped me tremendously not only with my weight issues but I have experienced first hand improvement in my personal and professional life as well as improvement in my relationships, my attitude, my mood and great financial gains as well.

Accept yourself today, just as you are, and start making the right choices to change the package you are in. Try reading, *Love Yourself and Let the Other Person Have It Your Way* by Lawrence Crane to help you do just that. You can download a free kindle version on Amazon. com.

VISUALIZATION

We often think of visualization in relation to meditation or prayer, but it can be a powerful tool in getting yourself mentally ready for the task of losing weight. Athletes often visualize themselves winning their race or the game before it even starts, because it helps them solidify their intentions. Picturing yourself getting stronger, thinner and more comfortable in your own skin will actually help you get there.

Visualization is not the same as using photos of yourself from when you are thinner, and I honestly don't recommend that technique. If you haven't been thin in a long time, you are older and heavier than what you were in that perfect picture from prom night or your wedding or in your favorite bikini. That was then and this is now – you aren't going to look like that photo again, you are going to look like something new: a better, stronger, thinner you! You don't want to look back when you visualize; you are creating the future by imagining what it looks like. It can be a very powerful experience. Spend some time with that vision. Focusing on that future you are planning for yourself can get you through some tough times.

GET SOME SUPPORT

Having a buddy to work out with or to lean on for support are the ideal conditions for losing weight. Many patients have come to me in tears because they are failing at losing weight. Once we start to talk about what's going on, I realize that they don't have their partner's support in getting healthy.

- Partner up: Whether it's your spouse, a good friend or a neighbor, find someone to exercise with, swap recipes with, and be a partner in losing weight. You will greatly increase your odds of succeeding if you have someone who will hold you accountable and pick you up when you fall.

- Go online: Your support can be virtual! There are tons of online support groups for weight loss and they are available 24 hours a day. Whatever your problem, you can find someone who has been through it.

- Find a group: A yoga studio, fitness center, YMCA or even your health care provider may organize weight-loss support groups in which people can come together and share success stories, obstacles and advice.

- Be your own cheerleader: Write some encouraging notes on the mirror, on the fridge or leave them in your car. Remind yourself why you are on this journey in the first place and that you can and will be successful.

Whatever type of support you find, be sure it is positive. You never want to lose weight to please someone else – your parents, your husband, and your kids. If someone is not being supportive of your efforts, do your best to tune that person out and replace his or her negativity with positive support. Every little bit counts when it comes to weight loss, and each time you make a good choice you are one step closer to your goal.

GET IN THE MOOD AND STAY THERE

You are in this for the long haul and you will need plenty of positive affirmations along the way.

You need to adopt a new outlook on your weight loss – that you are making changes toward a healthy lifestyle that will stay with you for good. You aren't depriving yourself of pizza and ice cream and chips; you are giving yourself the gift of a life full of vitality, health and happiness.

One way to keep the momentum going is to build a reward system into your diet. No, you won't be going out for a hot fudge sundae after a workout, but you can schedule things like manicures, spa appointments, shopping with friends or a movie night to celebrate milestones. Keep in mind that the scale can be fickle, even when you are working your hardest to keep its numbers going down. It will be much more gratifying to base your rewards on things like miles walked or the number of days you have been on your program rather than waiting for the scale to move to that next 10-pound mark.

Make the rewards frequent and fun to keep yourself focused on what great activity is coming up. Even when you are tempted to just cheat a little, you will have that extra incentive that you can get a pedicure in a few days if you just stay the course. If you have a diet buddy, you can help each other come up with rewards and enjoy them together – more reason to have them based on work rather than results; you can celebrate together.

When it comes to losing weight, your thoughts are powerful tools that you can use for good. Left unchecked, you may be sabotaging yourself at every turn rather than building up your store of support. If you need help, get it, and if you can help a friend, do it!

As I said in the beginning, I have been where you are today and I have helped my patients change their lives for the better. We are living in a culture that both demands we be thin and tempts us at every turn with foods and habits that would make us fat. If you want to be successful in your weight-loss goals, stick close to the ideas in this book, as they will serve you well. And, remember – it's not your fault that you are fat, but it will be up to you to make the change!

FOR MORE INFORMATION ON DETOX PRODUCTS, VITAMINS, WEIGHT LOSS AND HEALTH TIPS, VISIT THE WEBSITE WWW.ITSNOTYOURFAULTYOUREFAT.COM.

APPENDIX

Low-glycemic-index foods (less than 55)	GI
**Low-fat yogurt, sweetened	14
Peanuts	15
Artichokes	15
Asparagus	15
Broccoli	15
Cauliflower	15
Celery	15
Cucumber	15
Eggplant	15
Green Beans	15
Lettuce, all varieties	15
**Low-fat yogurt, artifically sweetened	15
Peppers, all varieties	15
Snow Peas	15
Spinach	15
Young summer squash	15
Tomatoes	15
Zucchini	15
Soy Beans, boiled	16
Cherries	22
Peas, dried	22
Milk, Chocolate	24
Pearl barley	25
Grapefruit	25
Milk, whole	27
Spaghetti, protein enriched	27
Kidney beans, boiled	29

Green lentils, boiled	29
Soy Milk	30
Apricots, dried	31
**Milk, skimmed	32
**Fettuccine	32
*M & M's (peanut)	32
Chickpeas	33
**Rye	34
**Milk, semi-skimmed	34
**Vermicelli	35
**Spaghetti. whole-wheat	37
Apples	38
Pears	38
Tomato soup, canned	38
Plums	39
**Ravioli, meat-filled	39
Carrots, cooked	39
*Snickers bar	40
**Apple Juice	41
**Wheat Kernels	41
**Spaghetti, white	41
Black-eyed peas	41
**All-Bran cereal	42
Peached	42
Chickpeas, canned	42
Oranges	44
Lentil soup, canned	44
**Carrot juice	45
**Maccaroni	45
**Pineapple juice	46
**Rice, instant	46
**Grapes	46

**Grapefruit juice	48
**Rice, boiled	48
**Multi-grain bread	48
**Baked beans, canned	48
**Oatmeal, instant	49
*Chocolate bar, 30g	49
**Jams and marmalades	49
**Whole grain	50
**Barley, cracked	50
*Ice-cream, lowfat	50
**Yams	51
**Orange Juice	52
Kidney beans, canned	52
Green lentils, canned	52
Kiwi fruit	53
*Pound Cake	54
**Bananas	54
Sweet Potatoes	54
*Potato chips	54

Notes: *high in empty calories, not recommended

Eating foods low on the glycemic index is a good general rule of thumb, however, the foods that are have * or ** are to be avoided, even though they are listed as low on the index.

Recommended Foods

PROTEIN

WILD SALMON
WILD COD
SARDINES

ORGANIC CHICKEN
SOLE
ORGANIC TURKEY
ORGANIC EGGS (RAW OR COOKED)
*IF YOU CANNOT FIND ORGANIC MEAT AT LEAST GET "NATURAL,"

VEGETABLES

AVOCADO
TOMATOES
EGGPLANT
PURPLE OR GREEN CABBAGE
MUSHROOMS
ARTICHOKES
ASPARAGUS
GREEN BEANS
BEETS
BROCCOLI
CAULIFLOWER
BROCCOLI RABE
BRUSSELS SPROUTS
CARROTS
CELERY
BUTTERNUT SQUASH
SPINACH
DARK, LEAFY GREENS
ROMAINE LETTUCE
BOSTON LETTUCE
RED-LEAF LETTUCE
ZUCCHINI
KALE
ONIONS
GARLIC
LEEKS
PARSNIPS
PEPPERS (ALL VARIETIES)
RADISHES
GINGER
CILANTRO
PARSLEY
DILL
GREEN ONIONS
BASIL

Add herbs such as cilantro, parsley, dill and basil for great flavor whenever possible.

Avoid potatoes (except in soup), sweet potatoes, rice, pasta and bread.

Notice peas and corn are not on the list, so avoid them at least for the first 30 days.

FRUITS

STRAWBERRIES
BLUEBERRIES
CRANBERRIES
POMEGRANATE
GOGI BERRIES
PINK GRAPEFRUIT
APPLES
PEARS
NECTARINES
PLUMS
PEACHES
AVOID BANANAS.

Preferably only one serving of fruit per day for the first 30 days.

DR. SONIA'S FAVORITE RECIPES

STUFFED EGGPLANT

1 LARGE EGGPLANT
2 CARROTS (GRATED)
1 SMALL PACKAGE BUTTON MUSHROOMS (CHOPPED)
½ WHITE ONION (CHOPPED)
2 CLOVES GARLIC (CHOPPED)
EXTRA VIRGIN OLIVE OIL
SEA SALT
PEPPER

SLICE THE EGGPLANT LENGTHWISE IN ¼-INCH-LONG STRIPS. PLACE ON A COOKIE SHEET AFTER BRUSHING EACH SIDE WITH EXTRA VIRGIN OLIVE OIL. SEASON LIGHTLY WITH SEA SALT AND FRESH GROUND PEPPER. BAKE IN THE OVEN FOR 20 MINUTES AT 350 DEGREES OR UNTIL SOFT. LET COOL. SAUTÉ CHOPPED ONIONS, MUSHROOMS AND GRATED CARROTS IN 2 TABLESPOONS OF EXTRA VIRGIN OLIVE OIL UNTIL SOFT. PLACE A LARGE SPOONFUL OF VEGETABLE MIXTURE ONTO EACH EGGPLANT STRIP AND ROLL EGGPLANT INTO LITTLE BUNDLES. (I OFTEN EAT THIS FOR BREAKFAST.)

CUCUMBER AND AVOCADO

6 SMALL CUCUMBERS
1 AVOCADO

CUT CUCUMBERS ON AN ANGLE INTO ¼-INCH SLICES (THEY'LL LOOKS LIKE CHIPS) AND ADD A SLICE OF AVOCADO WITH SOME SEA SALT. A GREAT SNACK THAT GIVES YOU THE CRUNCH OF NACHO CHIPS WITHOUT THE CARBS.

How to Make Any Vegetable Taste Good

Broccoli, cauliflower or other solid vegetable
Eggs (beaten)
Sea salt
Pepper
Extra virgin olive oil

Cut cauliflower and broccoli into small pieces (flowerettes). Dip in beaten egg. Add sea salt and pepper and lightly sauté in extra virgin olive oil. Very tasty.

Chicken Soup

6 chicken thighs
Sea salt
Pepper
3 carrots (grated or chopped)
1 cauliflower head
Cilantro
1 white onion
Parsley
Green onion
Garlic
1 can cannellini beans
2 red potatoes

Boil chicken in filtered water in a large soup pan. Season well with sea salt and pepper. A great seasoning is original Herbamare.

Then chop remaining fresh ingredients, add to chicken in pan and let it come to a boil. Turn down to a simmer for one hour. Rinse the beans in water and add at the very end when the soup is ready. It's simple and delicious. You don't even need any stock. Eat as much of this soup as you want as often as possible. I call it Diet Soup.

If you eat food bound to water you will feel more full and eat fewer calories. The only time potatoes are OK to eat is when they are in a soup.

SALAD DRESSING
JUICE OF 1 LEMON
JUICE OF 1 LIME
3 TBSPS. EXTRA VIRGIN OLIVE OIL
SALT
PEPPER

THIS IS ALL YOU NEED. IF YOU WANT TO GET FANCY, YOU CAN ADD CILANTRO AND PARSLEY WITH THE ABOVE INGREDIENTS IN A BLENDER. VERY FLAVORFUL, WITH NO SUGAR ADDED.

CHICKEN OR TURKEY BURGERS
1 LB. GROUND CHICKEN OR TURKEY (DARK MEAT); GRIND YOURSELF IF YOU CAN
1 BUNCH CILANTRO
1 BUNCH PARSLEY
3 GREEN ONIONS
2 ZUCCHINI (SHREDDED)
½ WHITE ONION
GARLIC
2 EGGS
SEA SALT
PEPPER
EGGS TO BIND

I PUT ALL OF THE ABOVE IN MY MEAT GRINDER. IF YOU DON'T HAVE A MEAT GRINDER, BUY THE MEAT ALREADY GROUND AND CHOP ALL INGREDIENTS (EXCEPT THE ZUCCHINI) INTO VERY TINY PIECES. GENTLY MIX ALL INGREDIENTS, INCLUDING SHREDDED ZUCCHINI, WITH THE EGGS AND FORM INTO LITTLE PATTIES. SAUTÉ IN EXTRA VIRGIN OLIVE OIL UNTIL COOKED THROUGH. YOU CAN ALSO SAUTÉ EACH SIDE FOR A FEW MINUTES AND FINISH BAKING IN THE OVEN AT 350 DEGREES.

(MAKE TWO OR THREE POUNDS AT A TIME IF YOU ARE ABLE. THEY FREEZE WELL AND LAST FOR ABOUT ONE WEEK IN THE FRIDGE.)

YOU CAN PUT THESE BURGERS IN A LEAF OF LETTUCE AND ADD PICKLE, TOMATO, ONION AND MUSTARD AND VOILA! A GREAT BURGER WITHOUT A BUN!

LASAGNA

6 ZUCCHINI
1½ LBS. GROUND TURKEY
1 JAR ORGANIC SPAGHETTI SAUCE, OR MAKE YOUR OWN
1 LARGE BUNCH OF SPINACH
ORGANIC MOZZARELLA (1 BAG SHREDDED)
½ WHITE ONION, CHOPPED SMALL
SALT
OLIVE OIL

SAUTÉ ONION AND BROWN GROUND TURKEY (I USE THE DARK MEAT FOR MORE FLAVOR AND TEXTURE). PUT OFF TO THE SIDE. CUT ZUCCHINI INTO VERY THIN STRIPS LENGTHWISE, USING A MANDARIN. SAUTÉ LIGHTLY WITH SALT AND OLIVE OIL, JUST ENOUGH TO GET THE WATER OUT. STEAM SPINACH AND ADD 1/8 CUP OF MOZZARELLA FROM THE BAG. USE ZUCCHINI LIKE YOU WOULD USE PASTA TO LAYER. PLACE 1/3 JAR OF SAUCE ON THE BOTTOM OF THE PAN, LAYER ZUCCHINI, THEN ADD MEAT LAYER, SPRINKLE WITH CHEESE, ADD 1/3 JAR OF SAUCE, ADD LAYER OF ZUCCHINI, SPREAD SPINACH AND CHEESE MIXTURE ON TOP, LAYER ZUCCHINI, 1/3 JAR SAUCE AND SPRINKLE WITH REMAINING CHEESE. COOK FOR 45 MINUTES UNTIL CHEESE BROWNS AND SAUCE IS BUBBLING.

ZUCCHINI PANCAKES

3 ZUCCHINIS
2 EGGS
SALT
PEPPER

OLIVE OIL

SHRED THE ZUCCHINI AND ADD EGGS. ADD SALT AND PEPPER TO TASTE. MAKE PATTIES AND SQUEEZE OUT EXTRA LIQUID. FRY IN OLIVE OIL.

TURKEY CHILI

1 LB. GROUND DARK TURKEY
1 CAN CANNELLINI BEANS
1 CAN KIDNEY BEANS
3 ZUCCHINI (CHOPPED)
2 CARROTS (CHOPPED)
2 JALAPENO PEPPERS (CHOPPED)
1 SERRANO PEPPER (CHOPPED)
1 RED PEPPER (CHOPPED)
2 GREEN PEPPERS (CHOPPED)
1 BUNCH PARSLEY (CHOPPED)
1 BUNCH CILANTRO (CHOPPED)
1 JAR WHOLE TOMATOES
1 LARGE WHITE ONION (CHOPPED)
3 CLOVES GARLIC (CHOPPED)
SALT
PEPPER

SAUTÉ ONION UNTIL SOFT. ADD TURKEY AND BREAK UP INTO FINE PIECES. ADD ALL THE VEGETABLES EXCEPT THE TOMATOES AND HERBS. COOK FOR 15 MINUTES. ADD TOMATOES AND HERBS AND SIMMER ON LOW FOR 15 MINUTES. ADD BEANS AND COOK FOR 5 MINUTES. THIS FREEZES VERY WELL AND WILL KEEP IN THE FRIDGE SO YOU CAN EAT ALL WEEK.

SALAD (I EAT THIS SALAD EVERY DAY!)

½ AVOCADO
BUNCH OF CILANTRO
15 GRAPE TOMATOES
6 KALAMATA OLIVES
¼ CUP RED ONION (SLICED)
¼ CUP CARROT (SHREDDED)
¼ CUP PURPLE CABBAGE (SHREDDED)
½ RED PEPPER (SLICED)
JUICE OF 1 LEMON
JUICE OF 1 LIME
OLIVE OIL
SALT
PEPPER

COMBINE ALL INGREDIENTS AND ADD THE LEMON AND LIME JUICE WITH A BIT OF OLIVE OIL. SALT AND PEPPER TO TASTE.

Royal Water

Add cucumbers, cilantro, mint, lemon or lime separately or in combination for a variety of delicious flavors.

This I discovered at the Royal Hotel spa when I was on vacation in Mexico. They had separate pitchers of cucumber water, mint water and lemon water.

Quesadilla Peppers (with no shells)

6 chicken pieces (can be breast, thighs, drumsticks, or even a whole chicken, preferably organic)
3 green peppers (can use red or yellow as well)
2 packages button mushrooms (chopped)
1 large white onion (sliced)
1 box organic no-chicken broth or use salted water
Salt
Pepper
Mozzarella for sprinkling

Boil chicken pieces in broth or water. Once chicken is cooked, remove from broth and let cool. Pick meat from bones with a fork and separate into thin strips. Cut peppers in half lengthwise and seed. Bake in the oven on a cookie sheet at 400 degrees until soft. Sauté onions and mushroom until soft. Add salt and pepper to taste. Add chicken to mushroom and onion mixture. Fill cooked halved peppers with chicken and vegetable mixture. Sprinkle with mozzarella cheese and bake at 400 degrees for 20-30 minutes or until cheese is brown and bubbling.

Green Soup

1 lb. ground dark turkey
1 tbsp. dried basil
1 tbsp. dried chives
1 tbsp. dried parsley
1 egg
1 large bag fresh green beans (chopped with ends removed)
3 zucchini (chopped)
½ bunch fresh parsley
½ bunch fresh cilantro
1 head broccoli (chopped)

1 BOX ORGANIC NO-CHICKEN BROTH
2 RED POTATOES (CHOPPED)
OLIVE OIL
SALT
PEPPER
1 LARGE WHITE ONION (CHOPPED)
2 CLOVES GARLIC (CHOPPED)

SAUTÉ ONION IN OLIVE OIL. ADD BROTH AND FILL SOUP POT 2/3 FULL OF WATER AFTER ADDING BROTH. ADD BROCCOLI, POTATOES, BEANS AND ZUCCHINI. ADD SALT AND PEPPER TO TASTE. SIMMER FOR 15 MINUTES ON MEDIUM.

MAKE MEATBALLS: PLACE GROUND TURKEY IN A BOWL, ADD SALT, PEPPER, DRIED HERBS AND EGG. MIX GENTLY WITH YOUR HANDS AND ROLL BETWEEN YOUR PALMS INTO LITTLE BALLS. TURN BURNER UNDER SOUP TO HIGH. DROP THE MEATBALLS INTO THE SOUP. BOIL ON HIGH FOR 10 MINUTES. ADD FRESH HERBS AND GARLIC TO TASTE.

(GREAT FOR KIDS, TOO; THEY LOVE MEATBALLS!)

OMELETS
BUTTER FOR PAN
BUTTON OR SHITAKE MUSHROOMS (HANDFUL)
2 GREEN ONIONS
3 EGGS
CREAM

BUTTER A SMALL PAN. ADD MUSHROOM AND GREEN ONIONS AND SAUTÉ UNTIL SOFT. IN A BOWL, BEAT THE EGGS WITH A SPLASH OF CREAM. ADD EGG MIXTURE TO FRYING PAN. ALLOW EGGS TO COOK ON THE BOTTOM AND THEN FOLD OVER. (YOU CAN ALSO JUST SCRAMBLE THE EGGS INTO THE MUSHROOMS.) AVOCADOS, SPINACH, BROCCOLI OR ANY VEGGIES WILL WORK FOR THIS RECIPE. EAT WITH HALF AN AVOCADO OR FRESH TOMATOES ON THE SIDE.

FISH IN TOMATO SAUCE

1-2 LBS. OF COD, CHOPPED INTO LARGE PIECES
2 CARROTS (SHREDDED)
1 LARGE WHITE ONION (CHOPPED)
1-2 TBSPS. TOMATO PASTE
OLIVE OIL
SALT
PEPPER
ORGANIC KETCHUP (JUST A LITTLE FOR A HINT OF SWEETNESS)

SAUTÉ CARROTS AND ONIONS IN OLIVE OIL WITH SALT AND PEPPER TO TASTE. POUR OVER CHOPPED FISH IN A LASAGNA PAN. IN A BOWL, MIX TOMATO PASTE, KETCHUP, ¼ CUP OF WATER, AND SALT AND PEPPER TO TASTE AND POUR OVER FISH. BAKE AT 350 DEGREES FOR 20-30 MINUTES UNTIL SAUCE BECOMES THICK AND WATER EVAPORATES.

AN ALTERNATIVE WOULD BE TO JUST BAKE THE FISH WITH THE CARROTS AND ONIONS UNTIL COOKED. ADD CHOPPED TOMATOES, ONIONS AND CILANTRO WITH LIME JUICE AND SALT AS TOPPING.

BEET SALAD

6 BEETS
3 CARROTS
½ JAR POLISH PICKLES OR ANY KIND YOU LIKE
½ WHITE ONION
DILL
LEMON

BOIL CARROTS AND ANY KIND OF BEETS UNTIL SOFT. PEEL AND CHOP INTO CUBES. ADD CHOPPED PICKLES, FINELY CHOPPED WHITE ONIONS, AND A HANDFUL OF CHOPPED DILL. SQUEEZE FRESH LEMON ON TOP. ADD SALT AND PEPPER TO TASTE. CHILL FOR 1 HOUR IN FRIDGE. SERVE COLD.

MOOD-ENHANCING SHAKE
1 CUP OF BERRIES (BLUEBERRIES, RASPBERRIES, STRAWBERRIES)
½ AVOCADO
2 ICE CUBES
2 TBSPS. GROUND FLAX SEEDS, PUMPKIN SEEDS, OR SUNFLOWER SEEDS
1-2 RAW EGGS
WATER

COMBINE INGREDIENTS IN A BLENDER. ADD WATER TO THIN SHAKE TO YOUR PREFERENCE. YOU WON'T EVEN TASTE THE EGGS. IF YOU CAN'T BRING YOURSELF TO EAT RAW EGGS, THEN LEAVE THEM OUT.

SUCCESS MENU FOR THE WEEK

(* note: drink hot water everyday before you eat breakfast)

	Breakfast	Lunch	Dinner
Monday	Strawberry, avocado and flax seed shake 1 glass hot water	Bowl of turkey chili	1 chicken breast 1 cup beet salad Dr. Sonia Salad
Tuesday	5 zucchini pancakes 1 glass hot water	2 chicken cutlet on lettuce leaves with pickles, tomatoes and mustard	1 large bowl chicken soup 1/2 Dr. Sonia Salad
Wednesday	Omelet 1/2 avocado 1 glass hot water	2 quesadilla peppers	Zucchini Lasagna (2 fist fulls)
Thursday	2 boiled eggs 1 cup home made juice or 1/2 avocado	1 stuffed eggplant 1 chicken thigh 1 cup beet salad	1 large bowl Green Soup Side of Cucumber
Friday	Spinach omelet Side of Fresh Tomatoes Glass hot water	1 cabbage salad 1 slice zucchini lasagna	Roasted Turkey Cauliflower in egg Brussel Sprouts
Saturday	Shake Hot water	Green Soup 1 stuffed eggplant	Eat Out! Follow the rules!
Sunday	Omelet Hot water 1/2 avocado	Turkey cutlets broccoli in egg Beet salad	Fish In Tomato sauce or salsa 1 Dr. Sonia Salad

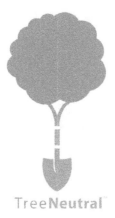

TreeNeutral

Printed in the USA
CPSIA information can be obtained
at www.ICGtesting.com
JSHW052018140824
68134JS00027B/2540